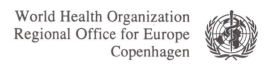

World Health Organization
Regional Office for Europe
Copenhagen

Health for all targets

The health policy for Europe

European Health for All Series, No. 4

ISBN 92 890 1311 7
ISSN 1012-7356

PRINTED IN FINLAND

Health for all targets

WHO Library Cataloguing in Publication Data

Health for all targets : the health policy for Europe

    (European health for all series ; No.4)

    1.Health for all 2.Health policy 3.Regional
    health planning I.Series

    ISBN 92 890 1311 7   (NLM Classification: WA 541)
    ISSN 1012-7356

Text editing: Pamela M. Charlton
Cover design: Sven Lund
Desktop layout: Wendy Enersen

CONTENTS

Foreword

"A blend of today's reality and tomorrow's dreams" was the vision the 32 Member States of the WHO European Region created in 1984 when they adopted the first set of European targets for health, an unprecedented act of solidarity and unity in the health field. That agreement did not come lightly. The whole idea that countries as different as those in the European Region would be able to agree on a common policy was met with disbelief by many. That politicians should stick their necks out, by clearly defining what levels of improvement they would try to reach within a given time, was abhorrent to those who felt that caution should always be paramount. After all, what would happen if a target was not reached – wouldn't someone be held accountable? With all the uncertainties of the future, how could anyone dare to estimate the target levels to aim for?

Nevertheless, as debate raged throughout the Region over the first draft of the targets sent to countries in 1983, the idea started to catch on. The draft was modified in the light of comments from Member States, and the second version was presented to the thirty-fourth session of the WHO Regional Committee for Europe in September 1984. Consensus had been created and the European health for all policy with its 38 targets was born.

What would follow? Would the voluminous document merely gather dust on a shelf, as so many other international agreements had done?

Today, nearly a decade later, we know that what began as a theoretical document on the agenda of the Regional Committee in 1984 has grown into a Region-wide movement that reaches into parliaments, government departments, city halls, the meetings of medical associations, the agendas of nursing associations, debates in pharmaceutical associations, development plans for schools of public health, the discussions of hospital administrators, the action plans of national diabetes associations, the research agendas of medical schools, the assistance programmes of intergovernmental organizations and elsewhere. Most important, local action deriving from the health for all policy has started directly to influence the lives of a steadily increasing portion of the 850 million people in the European Region. The European health *for all policy and targets have become a powerful public health movement in the Region.*

Why is this so? Health for all was not imposed by laws and regulations, nor did it lure countries, institutions or groups with financial incentives. It succeeded simply because its ideas proved to be sensible, practical and, above all, capable of inspiring people to think afresh, to take new initiatives and to work together in new ways. The policy's broad health agenda covers lifestyles, the environment and health services, addressing all levels of society and reaching out to all partners and sectors that can influence health. The health for all policy indicates very practical ways of stimulating better health development in the democratic, pluralistic societies of the Region today. Thus, it offers not only a vision of where to go for better health and quality of life but also a map showing how to get there. The policy used target setting at the international, national and local levels to communicate complex health goals to a wide range of groups and partners in countries, and established a system for monitoring progress towards the targets using specific indicators and a thorough evaluation at set intervals. Through these means, the health for all policy brought a new philosophy to the health development process in the countries of the Region. This open accountability forces countries, institutions and groups to measure the impact of political and administrative decisions on the health of the people, or on the performance of the systems that carry out interventions.

A cycle was established: target setting, implementation, monitoring, evaluation and the reformulation of targets and approaches. In this cycle, work for health for all becomes a continuous, natural learning process that ensures that people learn systematically from their successes and failures and – through

the international comparison permitted by WHO databases – from those of others.

And we need to learn! Although a Region-wide evaluation in 1991 showed that our progress is encouraging, the problems ahead are formidable. The most dramatic are the challenges facing the countries of the central and eastern part of the Region, not least a shortage of basic drugs and supplies. These countries' problems with health and health care do not differ in nature from those of the rest of the Region, but in degree and relative importance. All Member States must therefore take a similar approach to solving their problems.

Some 20 of the original 32 countries that made the European health for all policy in 1984 have used it as the framework for their own national health for all policies. Now the new democratic countries of the central and eastern part of the Region need to do the same. No other measure will help them so much to create a cohesive framework for development and to exploit all the resources for health that they must now muster in their present critical situation.

Problems are not confined to one part of the Region, however; all countries face a formidable challenge in helping their citizens choose healthier lifestyles, in improving the organization of their health services, in helping health professionals systematically to improve the quality of their care and in mobilizing societies to create healthier environments. Healthy environments mean not only freedom from the risks posed by pollution but also the creation of homes, neighbourhoods and cities that are safe and that promote health in a variety of ways, including the stimulation of personal interaction and support networks involving individuals, groups and communities.

Since the birth of the European movement for health for all, we have learned much from the action taken at all levels. There have been successes and failures; ideas have sprung up and new strategies been conceived and tested. Substantial progress has been made and many countries have already achieved a number of the European targets that were set for the year 2000.

Thus, the time came to take the European targets a major step forward, drawing on all our recent experience to formulate new levels or directions of achievement. The secretariat of the WHO Regional Office for Europe undertook the major task of revising the targets, with the help of hundreds of experts and the active and vital feedback of the Member States of the Region. This process reached its culmination at the forty-first session of the Regional Committee in Lisbon in 1991, at which the Member States updated the 1984 targets, retaining their framework and direction but adding the new elements, the new ideas and the new priorities that the Region now requires.

On behalf of the Regional Office, I extend warm thanks to all the countries, institutions and individuals who have participated in this task. The work has been carried out with an impressive degree of unity, a willingness to try new ideas from many sources and an ability to combine all the elements into a new whole.

The first book on the European targets was a best seller, translated into 19 languages and issued in many thousands of copies throughout the Region. May this version reach even further out and serve as an inspiration for many new initiatives throughout our continent – making today's reality into the tomorrow of our dreams!

J.E. Asvall
WHO Regional Director for Europe

1

The broad perspective

The European policy and targets for health for all unite the 850 million people in the Member States that constitute the European Region of WHO. This is an area whose borders are marked by the western shores of Greenland, the Mediterranean, and the Pacific shores of the Russian Federation. This book sets out the improvements in health that are sought by the year 2000, and describes the strategies for achieving them through healthier lifestyles, improvements in the environment and the provision of high quality services for prevention, treatment and care.

The desired improvement in health status and the factors that contribute to it are expressed as targets, some of which are quantified. The targets are intended to fuel the debate on health policies and their implementation in Member States. While not legally binding on any country, they express a collective commitment by Member States and provide help in setting targets that reflect the needs, priorities and values of different countries.

The new and revised targets incorporated in this book reflect changes that have taken place in the European Region since 1984 and a more up-to-date understanding of the problems involved in target setting and achievement. They are oriented towards the strategic action needed to achieve health for all.

The development of health for all and the first European targets The Thirtieth World Health Assembly laid the foundation for health for all in May 1977 when it decided that "the main social target of governments and WHO in the coming decades should be the attainment by all citizens of the world by the year 2000 of a level of health that will permit them to lead a socially and economically productive life" (resolution WHA30.43). This goal has global application and significance. Its particular relevance for the European Region is that, although considerable intellectual and financial resources have been invested, a great potential for health improvement remains and serious inequalities in health persist, both among Member States and among groups within individual countries.

In 1980, the thirtieth session of the Regional Committee for Europe met in Fez, Morocco, and approved the common European strategy for attaining health for all. The strategy called for fundamental changes in approaches to health development. It focused on four areas of concern: lifestyles and health, risk factors affecting health and the environment, the reorientation of the health care system, and the mobilization of political, managerial and technological support to bring about these changes. It also asked for a higher priority for health promotion and disease prevention, for positive steps by all sectors of society whose activities affect health, and for more emphasis on the role of individuals, families and communities. Improved primary health care was seen as the major approach to achieve these changes.

Years of working together in the Regional Committee had already demonstrated the common concern of Member States to improve the health and quality of life of their people. This history provided the background for the ambitious decision to formulate specific regional targets, despite the wide differences in social and economic conditions in the Region. Their successful formulation and their adoption by the thirty-fourth session of the Regional Committee in 1984 were decisive events that gave a strong impetus to the wide political acceptance and implementation of the European health for all strategy.

These events were a breakthrough in health development in the Region. For the first time, the Member States had agreed to adopt a single health policy as a common basis for individual and cooperative action. They also agreed to review their health situation and bring their policies and programmes in line with the health for all strategy. The process of implementation would be supported by systematic monitoring and reporting of progress every second year from 1983 onwards (subsequently changed to every third

year by resolution WHA39.7). The Regional Committee and World Health Assembly would consider the progress reports. In addition, the progress made would be evaluated every six years, beginning in 1985.

Progress and problems since 1985   Considerable progress has been made in several significant areas since the publication of the original targets in 1985. The concepts, principles and strategies of health for all have become widely reflected in national, regional and local policies and – most significant – the day-to-day health care practice throughout the Region. The monitoring and evaluation exercises that have taken place have deepened understanding of the progress made towards the achievement of health for all and the problems and dilemmas inherent in this process. The declarations, strategies and action plans that have come out of a number of WHO meetings have confirmed the strong relevance of the principles of health for all and clarified suitable approaches to their application.

Progress reports have shown the gains that have been achieved and the problems that remain. Life expectancy for the Region as a whole continues to increase and the overall maternal and infant mortality rates have dropped. Mortality rates for major diseases, including ischaemic heart disease, have fallen. Motor vehicle accidents occur less frequently. Transfrontier environmental pollution and hazardous wastes are more effectively controlled, and the quality of drinking-water has improved. Primary health care has become more widely available. The endorsement of health for all by all Member States and the development of health for all policies and strategies in nearly all countries of the Region have provided valuable support for this work.

Notwithstanding this progress, serious problems remain. Inequalities in health status between countries have not generally declined and in some cases they have increased, particularly between the countries in the central and eastern part of the Region and the rest. On average, cancer mortality is still increasing. Tobacco use, the excessive use of alcohol and the abuse of drugs continue to be serious lifestyle problems. Homicide and suicide are still too frequent. Progress in achieving cooperation between different sectors of government and with other sectors, such as private industry, in the interest of health has been disappointingly slow.

Specific lines of action Using the forum of WHO conferences, ministers of health and of related sectors have applied the principles and strategies of the European health policy to develop specific lines of action. The first European Conference on the Prevention and Control of Chronic Noncommunicable Diseases held in Varna, Bulgaria, in 1987 outlined future tasks, including further research in the field of prevention and control. A conference in Tbilisi, USSR, in 1990 analysed the relationship between inadequate family planning services and the high number of abortions and adopted the Tbilisi Declaration, which deals broadly with this problem area.

An international conference on health promotion, held in Ottawa in 1986, considered lifestyles conducive to health and produced the Ottawa Charter for Health Promotion. The Charter outlines a comprehensive strategy for health promotion with five dimensions: healthy public policy, supportive environments, personal skills, community action and reoriented health services. It reaches beyond traditional health services with broader terms of reference, putting more emphasis on health as opposed to illness and creating a different relationship with the community. A second international conference on health promotion, focusing on healthy public policy, was held in Adelaide, Australia, in 1988 and a third on supportive environments for health in Sundsvall, Sweden, in 1991.

The first European Conference on Tobacco Policy, held in Madrid in 1988, developed a plan of action that had as its foundation the aim of promoting nonsmoking as the norm in Europe. The first European Conference on Food and Nutrition Policy was held in Budapest in 1990 to establish the groundwork for national food policies and action plans that would be sensitive to nutritional issues.

Strong concern about health issues in the environment led to the unanimous adoption of the European Charter on Environment and Health by 29 Member States and the Commission of the European Communities, at the First European Conference on Environment and Health held in Frankfurt in 1989. The Charter sets out predictive and preventive strategies that will reverse negative trends in the quality of the environment and will improve living conditions and increase wellbeing. It defines the entitlements and responsibilities of individuals, as well as public and private organizations. It emphasizes the implementation of policy by identifying strategies and priorities for prevention, management and control.

Addressing the development of appropriate services, the first European Conference on Nursing, held in Vienna in 1988, defined the need for a new type of primary health care nurse at the community level.

Finally, to mobilize support for health for all, a European Conference on Planning and Management for Health, held in The Hague in 1984, developed a new concept of health planning and made a breakthrough in thinking on how health for all developments could be stimulated in the pluralistic societies of the Region today. Following the Edinburgh Declaration at the World Conference on Medical Education in 1988, European ministers of health and of education met in Lisbon at the Ministerial Consultation for Medical Education in Europe. They adopted the Lisbon Initiative, which states that medical education in the Region should from now on be based on the European health for all policy and the principles of the Edinburgh Declaration.

Updating the targets   The original target book set 1990 as the achievement date for more than half the targets. This, together with the widespread changes that have taken place in the Region since 1984, meant that the targets needed updating. In 1989, the Consultative Group on Programme Development (CGPD) and the Regional Committee at its thirty-ninth session decided that an update was timely, but that the basic structure of the target book should be retained and only necessary changes introduced. Views and guidance on the updating were obtained through a questionnaire sent to Member States in 1989. An epidemiological review was carried out to supplement the results of the 1988 health for all monitoring exercise, and a consultation on future trends in society was held early in 1990. The Regional Health Development Advisory Council (RHDAC) then held a brainstorming session on target updating. The fortieth session of the Regional Committee endorsed all these preparatory activities. In 1991, the CGPD and an informal consultation on updating the European regional targets for health for all made further suggestions on the content of the update document.

Based on all these different inputs, the targets were revised and an updated set of targets was approved at the forty-first session of the Regional Committee in 1991.

As in 1984, the underlying aim of the updating has been to set targets that are "a blend of today's reality and tomorrow's dreams". The formulation of targets varies according to the nature of the problem they address and the extent of knowledge available on the existing situation. The levels set for quantified targets are not the result of elaborate mathematical modelling, but are based on historical trends, analysis and expected future evolution.

The base year for the targets remains 1980, and the year 2000 is now the completion date for all of them. In other words, the targets have become a description of the state of health, the factors contributing to health, the health policy, and the lines of action desired at the end of this century. For reference, the relationship between the subjects dealt with in the updated targets and the 1984 targets is shown in Annex 1.

In the 1985 target book, indicators were included to provide the basis for systematic monitoring and evaluation of progress in each Member State and in the Region as a whole. Member States have used them in reporting progress to WHO in 1985, 1988 and 1991. The indicators were revised in 1988 in the light of experience up to that point. Additional revisions have been made to reflect the reformulation of targets that has taken place (Annex 2). A plan of action has also been revised (Annex 3), indicating the major steps that Member States and WHO will take in cooperation to monitor and evaluate their progress towards the targets and, ultimately, to update the targets further to bring them into the twenty-first century. The revised indicators and plan of action were approved at the forty-first session of the Regional Committee in 1991.

Status of the targets The updated targets indicate the improvements that could be expected if all the will, knowledge, resources and technology already available were pooled in pursuit of common goals. The targets represent the joint aspiration of all the Member States of the European Region, an aspiration that will inspire and motivate them when they are setting their own targets and priorities and assessing their own capacities. The means used to reach each target are the responsibility of individual Member States, taking into account their political, legal, social and economic positions and the practicalities of their health systems and organizational structures.

Content and structure of this book The remainder of this section introduces the contents of the different chapters and targets and their interrelationships.

Chapter 1 concludes by identifying the major themes of the European health for all policy that are essentially the values and principles that underlie the targets.

Chapter 2 deals with the changing social, political and economic situation in the Region, and discusses the prerequisites for health. Since 1984, remarkable changes have taken place. The population has grown older and the structure of family life has changed. Concern about the environment and its effects on health has grown rapidly. Unprecedented political and economic developments have occurred in the central and eastern part of the Region, and the evolution of European integration

has continued. These trends are discussed and their implications for the future of health are explored.

Fig. 1 gives a brief overview of the content and structure of the target chapters (3 – 7). The health outcomes that are sought through the application of the health for all strategy in the European Region are the subject of Chapter 3 (targets 1 – 12). Targets 1 – 12 express in specific and, where possible, quantified terms the improvements in health status sought over the 20 years between the Regional Committee approval of the health for all strategy in 1980 and the year 2000.

These health outcomes have four interrelated themes, which are woven throughout the 12 targets:

- *ensuring equity in health* by reducing gaps in health status between countries and between groups within countries;
- *adding life to years* by helping people achieve, and use, their full physical, mental and social potential;
- *adding health to life* by reducing disease and disability;
- *adding years to life* by increasing life expectancy.

The first 12 targets fall into three categories: the basic health for all goals, the health of vulnerable populations and specific health problems. These targets set the objectives and agenda for the three chapters (4 – 6) that follow, which address the changes in lifestyles, the improvements in the environment, and the developments in prevention, treatment and care that will make their achievement possible.

Chapters 4, 5 and 6 address the main strategies for achieving health for all. Chapter 4 (targets 13 – 17)

Fig. 1. The health for all targets

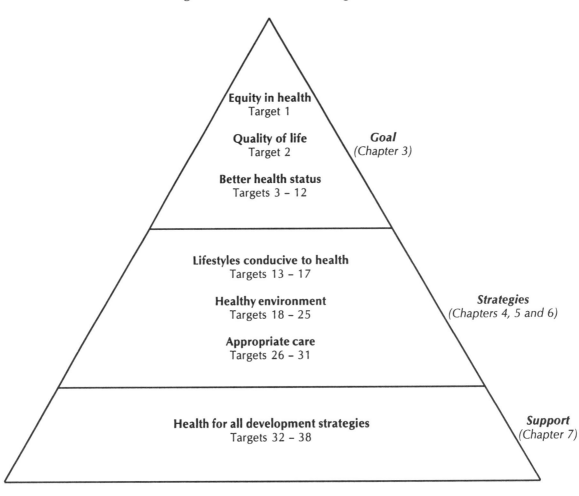

addresses the health work that is essential to attain lifestyles conducive to health. It relies on the principles expressed in the 1986 Ottawa Charter for Health Promotion. It proposes national, regional and local initiatives that actively support healthy patterns of living, such as balanced nutrition and appropriate physical activity, and reductions in the health-damaging consumption of substances such as alcohol and tobacco. While fully recognizing the value of improving people's knowledge of and motivation for health through health education, the health for all policy gives major emphasis to changes in the social, economic, cultural, physical and other factors that influence the health-related choices made by individuals, groups and communities. It therefore stresses the importance of intersectoral action as a basis for strengthening the opportunities for health promotion in all settings of life such as cities, places of work, schools and homes.

Chapter 5 (targets 18 – 25) is concerned with the contribution of the environment to health and draws on the philosophy and strategies of the European Charter on Environment and Health and on the report of the World Commission on Environment and Development.[a] It reflects the emerging commitment to environmental policies that lead to ecologically sustainable development, the prevention and control of risks, and equitable access to healthy environments. The targets' aim is to provide opportunities for people to live in communities with socially and physically supportive environments.

Chapter 6 (targets 26 – 31) addresses the provision of appropriate services for prevention, treatment and care. Locally accessible primary health care is the focus of the chapter, supported by secondary and tertiary care that is comprehensive and responsive to health needs, and supplemented by services for people with special needs. A central theme of the chapter is the effective management of human, financial and physical resources in a manner that is consistent with the development of cost-effective services of quality.

The interventions proposed in Chapters 4, 5 and 6 require sustained political, managerial and financial support and mobilization, linked together through an infrastructure that allows a coordinated approach to policy formulation and implementation. These are the subjects of Chapter 7 (targets 32 – 38). The foundation for health for all development is the formulation of a health policy and an implementation strategy that take a balanced approach to the subject areas of health

for all and rest on strong political accountability at different levels. The targets in Chapter 7 emphasize how important it is for institutions to inspire, mobilize and guide health development, to facilitate intersectoral cooperation and community participation, and to manage human resource development. The chapter also deals with the research and information support necessary for health for all development, as well as the need to develop appropriate mechanisms to strengthen ethical considerations in decisions relating to health.

The targets set out in Chapters 3 to 7 are closely interrelated. The relationships between targets within each chapter are illustrated in the introductory sections. More detailed connections, within and between chapters, are discussed in the sections on individual targets.

Chapter 8 is the final chapter in the book. It brings together some conclusions about the European health for all policy and some challenges and problems facing its implementation. It also picks up the theme of the interconnectedness of the targets in a different way, by illustrating how taking action on health for all does not mean tackling targets one by one. Different components of the targets can be combined into cohesive programmes of action – the example given is of a potential programme of action on tobacco that combines components from many different targets.

Major themes of the European health policy The first target book identified six major themes that ran through the whole document. These remain equally relevant in this revised book, but to them must be added a seventh, a concern with ethics. Although this is implicit in the first target book, only now does it find explicit

---

[a] WORLD COMMISSION ON ENVIRONMENT AND DEVELOPMENT. *Our common future*. Oxford, Oxford University Press, 1987.

recognition through the commitment in the new target 38 to take into account ethical considerations in all decisions relating to health. The seven themes set out below are essentially the values and principles that underlie all 38 targets and the European health policy they express.

- *Equity* is the essence of health for all. Equity in health means that all people have a fair opportunity to realize their full health potential. It requires action to reduce inequalities in health status between and within countries. Equity policies involve improving the living and working conditions of the disadvantaged, so as to raise the standards of their physical and social environment to levels closer to those of more fortunate groups.

- The concern with *ethics* is a new theme reflected throughout this book. The basic principle of equity can be seen as a reflection of a profound concern for ethics. Ethical issues arise throughout all arenas in the health sector – in health policy, in connection with the rights of individuals, groups of patients and whole communities, and in connection with specific health care interventions – as well as in connection with the intersectoral policies and actions that are required for the achievement of health for all. The European health policy seeks appropriate mechanisms to strengthen ethical considerations in all decisions relating to the health of individuals, groups and populations.

- People themselves will achieve health for all. Well informed and well motivated, actively *participating communities* are key elements in setting priorities, and in making and implementing decisions. This approach makes the best use of existing human resources while strengthening individual self-worth and knowledge and encouraging the provision of social support.

- The main emphasis of health policy and strategy is on *health promotion* and *disease prevention*. This gives people a positive sense of health so that they can make full use of their physical, mental and social capacities. This emphasis needs to be reflected in the promotion of positive lifestyles, the building of supportive environments and the reorientation of health services.

- *Primary health care* should be the focus of the health service system. This means meeting the basic health needs of each community through services that are located as close as possible to where people live and work, are easily accessible, and involve the community in their development, planning and implementation.

- Many sectors of society need to collaborate in the achievement of health for all. *Intersectoral action* is needed to ensure access to the prerequisites for health and protection from risks in the physical, economic and social environment. Such action implies cooperation among agencies of government at the national, regional and local levels and with other sectors such as business and industry, labour unions and professional groups. It also implies a constant search for quality and cost-effectiveness.

- An increasing number of health problems transcend national frontiers. Strong *international cooperation* is required to ensure environmental protection, access to adequate resources for healthy living, and the provision of care that is of high quality and takes the best advantage of current knowledge and technology.

The future The targets presented in this book maintain the effort to change the course of health development in the Region that started with the first target book. What is at stake is ultimately the health and wellbeing of the Region's children, of the coming generations. The success of the health for all movement will mean that all children of the Region will have a much better chance of:

– being born healthy to parents who want them and who have the time, the means and the skills needed to bring them up and care for them properly;
– being educated in societies that endorse the basic values of healthy living, encourage individual choice and allow it to be exercised freely;

– being provided with the basic requirements for health and being effectively protected against disease and accidents.

It also means that all people would have an equal opportunity of:

– living in a stimulating environment of social interaction, free from the risk of war or civil conflict, with full opportunities for playing satisfying economic and social roles;
– growing old in a society that supports the maintenance of their capacities, provides for a secure, purposeful retirement, offers care when care is needed and, finally, allows them to die with dignity.

2

The future of health in the European Region

Opportunity and challenge Since the adoption of the original regional targets in 1984, political developments have had profound effects on the social fabric and the conduct of public affairs in all parts of the Region. The ending of the Cold War and of its sterile ideological divide in the Region means that issues of public policy for health can now be discussed openly and ideas and experience freely exchanged. The impetus for political and economic change in the central and eastern part of the Region continues as these countries move towards a pluralistic democracy and a market economy. The evolution in western and southern Europe of the European Community, and the possible eventual creation of a wider European economic, social and political entity, will necessitate cooperation, openness and flexibility throughout the Region.

Concomitant with the geopolitical and economic transformations, the Region has been going through a phase of technological innovation and rapid social change that has serious health consequences. The effects of change demonstrate the importance of both international cooperation and a sound public health infrastructure in all Member States. Growing attention to the relationships between health, environment and economic development underscores the point. The protection and promotion of health require an environment in which physical, social and psychological factors are all given due importance. Environmental standards need to be continually reviewed to take account of new knowledge about the relationships between the environment, economic development and health. Environmental problems do not halt at national borders and their resolution requires an ecological health policy and intersectoral action at the international level.

The European Charter on Environment and Health, adopted at Frankfurt in 1989, highlighted issues requiring urgent action at local, national and international levels. These include global disturbances to the environment, such as the destruction of the ozone layer and climatic change; safe and adequate drinking-water supplies with hygienic waste disposal for all urban and rural communities; the microbiological and chemical safety of food; the impact on the environment and on health of various energy options, of transport, especially road transport, and of agricultural practices, including the use of fertilizers and pesticides; the quality of air, especially in relation to oxides of sulfur and nitrogen; and the quality of indoor air (residential, recreational and occupational) including the effects of radon, passive smoking and chemicals.

The Charter also drew attention to the management and disposal of hazardous wastes, to the need for contingency planning for accidents and disasters, and to the health aspects of urban development and renewal. The opening of national borders across the Region and the speedier flow of goods and information could well affect lifestyles and health behaviour. A comprehensive and coherent approach to health protection and promotion is therefore clearly needed, encompassing both human behaviour and environmental factors.

Research and development leading to advances in medical and related technology, including genetic engineering, will result in new and better options for prevention, treatment, rehabilitation and nursing care. Some of the advances also raise difficult ethical issues, however, which need to be debated since they often concern matters of life and death and pose policy questions about the use of limited health resources. Coincidentally, continuing developments in information technology will lead to better information support for health policy and decision-making at all levels, thereby enhancing the quality of policy development in Member States and the efficiency of its implementation.

Information technology will also facilitate WHO's task as a clearing-house for the exchange of information and ideas in support of policy and practice within Member States. One consequence of geopolitical change is that the European Region now comprises over 50 Member States. Some of the new states will be small and will need particular support. Many will need help to develop democratic practices in policy-making and implementation and specifically to strengthen their public health infrastructures.

Possible futures   The relevance for the 1990s of the updated European targets can be seen very clearly by putting them in the context of a number of possible trends in a future Europe. These are not predictions, but could all be plausible on the basis of what is already known.

Despite certain current difficulties facing Member States, some underlying trends point towards improved economic performance. In particular, greater intercountry economic cooperation should create more favourable conditions for growth in Member States. Systematic development assistance from the international community will be a forceful stimulus for the restructuring and expansion of the economies of the countries in the central and eastern part of the Region. This assistance will protect those countries from the full consequences of the transition from their previous economies, and thereby stabilize the Region as a whole.

The equitable distribution of the results of improved economic performance should lead to greater material wellbeing and an associated health gain for all. An alternative possibility, however, is that, even with an economic upturn, inequity in health will increase through widening differences between socioeconomic groups and also between affluent regions and economically backward ones. The widest gap could be between the employed, particularly those with skills in strong demand, and the unemployed who lack those skills, as well as the apparently unemployable, disabled and other socially disadvantaged groups. Long-term unemployment will have a particularly negative effect on health where there is little experience of how to alleviate its worst socioeconomic and psychological effects. The downward social and economic mobility of those who have previously lived in secure material circumstances will also be detrimental to health, and the numbers of these so-called new poor are likely to grow. Health may also be adversely affected by continued mobility and the splitting up of family structures, further urbanization through drift from the rural areas, and changes in social security systems that limit benefits.

Migration will increase both from outside the Region, by people seeking greater economic opportunities, and from within, by people moving to more affluent areas. Flows will mainly be from east to west and south to north, with tourism in the opposite directions. Migration carries both positive and negative health and social consequences for the migrants and the host community. One particular risk might be social and political pressures to distinguish between the rights of the indigenous population who have citizen status and those of migrants. The health consequences of these movements have both intersectoral and international significance.

The shape of the population pyramid in the Region has changed markedly this century and will change further in coming decades. Europeans already enjoy a longer life span than the peoples of any other region in the world, and it is still lengthening. The number of the very old, that is people over 80 years of age, will increase considerably. They have far more health problems and disabilities than younger age groups, which will mean a corresponding increase in the need for health and social services for this population. In the past the children, particularly

daughters, of the frail and dependent elderly have acted as "cover carers" for their parents. In future, for various social and economic reasons, women may be less likely to forego paid employment to care for relatives. Even families retaining strong emotional ties may be scattered geographically. A particular difficulty can arise when the children of the very old themselves start to experience the health and mobility problems associated with aging and are increasingly unable to fulfil what would have been an expected and welcome role. The health and social policy implications of the needs of the very old and the adequacy and quality of the services they receive, or should receive, are matters requiring close scrutiny.

At the same time, the active group of the third age is growing. Spanning late middle-age to the mid or late 60s, this group includes people who have retired from their regular occupations and who have long since fulfilled their family commitments as child rearers. They are physically fit and psychologically ready for stimulus and challenge. They have many years of active retirement in front of them, but today they receive very little recognition except from the leisure industry. Public policy and the social system will need to mobilize this group, so that its members can fully realize their potential contribution to society.

Higher educational levels and greater sophistication will lead patients and other users of health and social services to demand more choice and participation. This trend will stimulate a better quality of care and encourage the emergence of new professional attitudes towards the users of services. It should also result in a greater commitment to the reallocation of health sector resources, and a review of the education of health professionals leading to a more comprehensive understanding of the health needs of a community.

Further, whatever the macroeconomic trends in the Region, the pressures on health sector resources, whether driven by demographic, technological or other forces, will continue if not intensify. Conscious efforts will be required to achieve a more equitable distribution of limited resources, better management and greater efficiency in performance.

The most positive projections for the future describe a society that will become more responsible, cooperative and caring. Increasing political, economic and social convergence will foster agreement to tackle urgent transboundary health problems. Local communities will be the workshops for making living and working environments more healthy. Equality between the sexes will increase, with mutual respect and support. Technological and economic changes will see not only a reduction of working hours but the creation of new forms of social organization, including those that share the burden of care of the growing number of people who will need various forms of assistance. While the activities of voluntary and mutual support groups may often need to be underpinned by effective public services, this trend towards self-help certainly warrants reinforcement by health policy.

In this scenario, work will still be a very important source of personal identity, but each individual's participation in the labour market will have greater flexibility. Acquiring the education, knowledge and skills to be applied at work will be seen as a life-long endeavour, not as confined to adolescence and early adulthood. Society will abandon fixed expectations of the behaviour of individuals and groups occupying various social roles. It will be ready to accept a wider variety of cultural differences and a multitude of different lifestyles, and will expect constructive social and political outcomes from the interaction between different groups.

None of these trends and projections can be expected to work out exactly as they have been introduced here. Much will depend on how the political trend of the 1980s of applying market principles to all forms of social organization ultimately works out in the 1990s. Public policy may come to be seen in terms that narrow the range of issues on the political agenda to those minimizing public spending and redefining collective rights. Nevertheless, the emphasis on individual responsibility and opportunities for economic self-advancement need not necessarily replace the values of solidarity, mutual support and collective action that were originally behind the creation of the twentieth-century welfare state.

It will therefore be important to continue to debate the issues covered in this sketch of possible futures. Further national and international research and trend analysis can build up a sound base of evidence on which crucial decisions affecting the people of the Region can be made. This should ensure that political debate is not limited to strategies for economic growth, but also focuses on people's health and the quality of their lives.

Prerequisites for health   The Region's current trends will not alter the basic nature of countries' health development needs, and the fundamentals of the European health for all strategy will therefore remain as relevant in the year 2000 as they are in 1993, and indeed were in 1980 when the strategy was first formulated: to prevent and control disease, to promote and maintain health, to ensure a healthy environment, and to provide health services appropriate to people's needs. The regional targets are a reflection of present and anticipated trends, perceived problems and known resources and technology.

Much still has to be done to prevent disease and disability, to create the conditions for healthy living and to make health care more responsive to people's needs. Such improvements as are achieved will not have their full effect, however, if certain prerequisites for health are not met. The main political responsibility for securing these prerequisites falls on governments, but the challenge must be taken up at all levels of policy-making within countries. All public bodies and private sector organizations and enterprises have a part to play, since their decisions and actions address those aspects of life that are prerequisites for the health of their voters, customers and clients.

Peace   War remains the most serious of all threats to health. The devastation that a war entails, whether in terms of the people killed, wounded, permanently disabled and displaced from their homes and communities, or of its impact on the environment, is well understood. The health argument against nuclear war has been forcefully debated in recent years. It must not be forgotten, however, that hostilities within countries and so-called conventional war are also terrible threats to humanity. The 1991 Gulf hostilities and their aftermath have very clearly demonstrated the results of a major international armed conflict. In 1992 – 1993, fighting has brought terrible suffering to millions of people in the Region, especially in former Yugoslavia and the former Soviet Union.

The nuclear threat and Cold War assumptions no longer shape geopolitics. The end to the old forms of international tension in the Region promises new opportunities for all its peoples to work together in harmony for a better future. It is disappointing, therefore, that the movement towards independence in some parts of the Region has been accompanied by armed conflict. In addition, there is concern that the improvement in international relations may be offset by the renewal of deep-seated but hitherto suppressed antagonisms between ethnic and religious groups, both in their own and other countries. Moreover, conflicts between such groups and controversies between immigrants and local populations may increase as a result of the opening of borders, especially in areas experiencing serious economic problems.

Peace is not just the absence of war. It cannot be called peace if civil unrest and ethnic conflict continue to erupt into violence and armed struggle as they do in some countries. As threats to health, these forms of aggression are scarcely less serious than war itself, in the psychological trauma that comes from living in fear of violence, in the effects of intentional injury and post-trauma distress syndrome such as suffered by torture victims, and in the indirect effects of long-term damage to the social, physical and economic structures of the countries and communities affected.

Peace is, like health itself, a positive sense of wellbeing and security, implying the opportunity for all to develop to the full their own human potential. It assumes the possibility that all countries can participate actively on a basis of solidarity and reciprocity in the development of a more stimulating and satisfying world for their populations.

The health sector should continue to do whatever both fits in with its basic role and can help to promote harmony and reduce international tension. In each country, the health sector should continue to take the lead in fostering close, long-term collaboration on health problems across national borders. The bilateral and international research, meetings and contacts involved, in addition to improving health, will increase understanding and forge links between individuals, institutions and countries, thus demonstrating the value of mutual cooperation.

Equity in health and the satisfaction of basic needs   In the commitment to health for all lies the fundamental principle of equity. This means that all human beings have the right to equal opportunities to develop and sustain their full health potential. This principle has two aspects: equity among nations and equity among the people within each country. Very large differences in standards of living remain between the countries of the Region. These differences in socioeconomic development translate into disturbing inequalities in health status. The increased flow of information on these matters, particularly from the countries in the central and eastern part of the Region, has given a clear picture of the sharp contrasts in health status and in access to health services between and within countries of the Region.

Pockets of social and economic deprivation are often found in the more developed countries of the European Region. Life expectancy is lower and infant mortality is higher in these disadvantaged socioeconomic groups than in the rest of the population. Various such disadvantaged groups have been identified, such as very old people, refugees and immigrants, members of ethnic minorities, people living in specific deprived geographical areas, and single parent families reliant on either low wages or state benefits. The numbers in these groups are likely to grow in countries facing economic difficulties and the dislocations of political change.

A major task in any national policy-making, if it is to be consonant with health for all values, must be the establishment of a consistent and long-term strategy capable of attacking the causes of social inequity. It must address the problems of insufficient disposable income to satisfy basic needs such as food, good nutrition and decent housing, the lack of neighbourhood amenities including sanitation and safe drinking-water, and poor education and employment opportunities. The targets should be seen as proposing the health component of a national social policy to reduce inequity.

Political will and public support   Today's challenges mean that health has to be seen as a responsibility not only of the health sector but also of other sectors – whether they be education, media, transport, agriculture, industry or others. The Ottawa Charter for Health Promotion and the European Charter on Environment and Health both reinforce this basic strategic intent of health for all. Strong political will and the mobilization of public support are needed to ensure that the necessary action is taken. The process of sustaining and mobilizing further support should be seen as a national responsibility at the highest level and pursued in all sectors throughout the country. Ministries of health, together with other health authorities and private and professional bodies, should act in concert to sustain commitment to the values as well as the target objectives of health for all.

Precisely how people are mobilized depends on the cultural and social patterns and the constitutional and political structures in the country concerned. Nevertheless, mobilization involves engaging the active support of civic and religious leaders and other public figures, such as those representing business, trade unions and influential non-governmental organizations in all sectors of society. Continuing efforts must be made to ensure that the health professions, various social groups and particularly community organizations become and remain active collaborators in pursuing health for all objectives. The experience of engaging all these groups in the broad health for all movement over the past decade suggests that the effort to mobilize their support pays its own dividend.

International cooperation   The strong, collective political commitment of Member States is essential to maintain the impetus for the action required by the regional targets. Resolutions adopted by the United Nations General Assembly and the World Health Assembly call on countries to develop their own health for all strategies and take the necessary steps to ensure their implementation.

A key problem for the less developed countries of the Region is a lack of investment and inadequate development in the health sector. A major challenge for the European Region, therefore, is how to secure and sustain concrete forms of solidarity that enable the more developed countries to offer effective support and collaboration to those less well provided for, thus ensuring the rapid development of their health sectors. Solidarity of this sort was shown in the 1980s when the countries of the Region helped to promote and support the rational development of comprehensive health care systems in southern European countries. Another significant and timely indication of regional solidarity was the initiative taken by the Regional Committee in 1990 to create a regional programme, EUROHEALTH, to intensify cooperation in health with the countries of central and eastern Europe. The programme is designed to help these countries reform and strengthen their health care systems and base their health policies on health for all values. Its greatest potential lies in its coordination with the European Community's PHARE programme (on aid for economic restructuring in countries of central and eastern Europe), the Council of Europe's DEMOSTHENE programme (to promote fellowships in those countries) and the WHO/UNICEF aid programme to the Commonwealth of Independent States.

The Regional Committee, by its continuing interest in the periodic health for all monitoring and evaluation exercises, and individual Member States, by their readiness to report and share their experience and achievements, have sustained their commitment. The updating of the targets now is the strongest possible message to all concerned that health for all values remain relevant to Member States and their commitment to it remains as clear as ever.

3

Achieving better health

The twelve targets in this chapter describe the desired health outcomes of the health for all strategy in the European Region. They set out the improvements in health status that the Regional Committee approved in the health for all strategy in 1980 and that remain the goal for the year 2000. These targets set the agenda for the three subsequent chapters, which address the changes in lifestyles, the environmental improvements and the developments in prevention, treatment and care that will make these outcomes possible.

The outcome targets can be grouped into three different categories (see Fig. 2) reflecting different concerns within public health. These are the basic health for all goals, the health of vulnerable population groups, and specific health problems. Chapter 3 provides a framework for comprehensive policy development, planning and implementation to support each target. Details of the policies and implementation measures required to achieve the targets in this chapter are taken up in the next three chapters.

The main concern in Chapter 3 is strategy. The strategies suggested all rely heavily on improved access to the prerequisites for health such as food, shelter and income, the creation of safe and supportive physical and social environments, opportunities to lead healthy lifestyles and easy access to primary health care. The unique quality of strategies based on equity is that they must be particularly responsive to the needs of the disadvantaged.

The health for all goal The first category comprises two targets concerned with the basic policy orientation of the European health for all strategy: the achievement of equity in health and the improvement of health and quality of life.

The health of vulnerable groups The second category contains four targets (of which three have a new focus) concerned with the health of particular population groups: people with disabilities, children and young people, women, and the elderly. Three considerations have influenced the selection of these groups as requiring special attention: the people in each of these groups often

Fig. 2. The goal: achieving better health

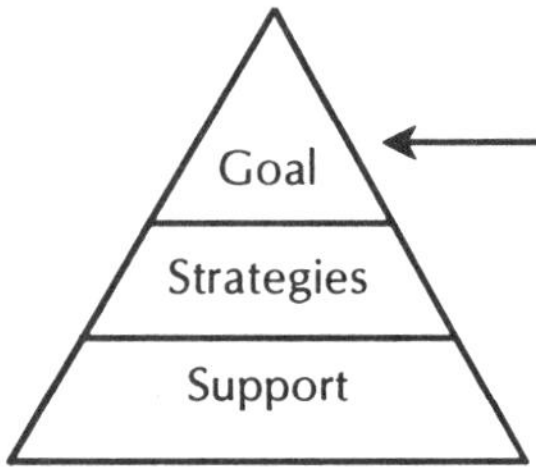

Goal

Strategies

Support

Fig. 1

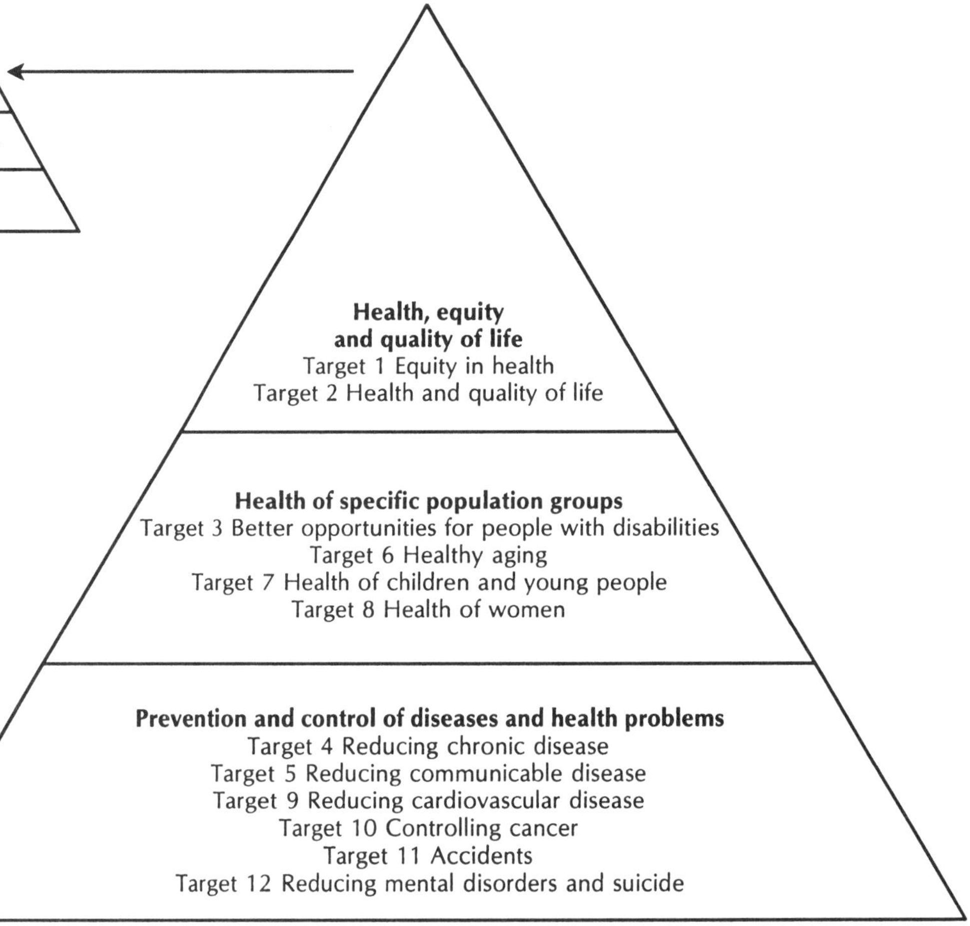

**Health, equity
and quality of life**
Target 1 Equity in health
Target 2 Health and quality of life

Health of specific population groups
Target 3 Better opportunities for people with disabilities
Target 6 Healthy aging
Target 7 Health of children and young people
Target 8 Health of women

Prevention and control of diseases and health problems
Target 4 Reducing chronic disease
Target 5 Reducing communicable disease
Target 9 Reducing cardiovascular disease
Target 10 Controlling cancer
Target 11 Accidents
Target 12 Reducing mental disorders and suicide

suffer a relative disadvantage in terms of their health and social status; they have specific health needs; and they can benefit from the implementation of strategies that add life to years by emphasizing intersectoral approaches.

Specific health problems   The third category consists of six targets concerned with specific health problems: cancer, cardiovascular disease, other chronic diseases, communicable disease, accidents, and mental disorders and suicide. They have much in common in terms of strategic perspective and policy development. Common themes within the targets in this category include a concern with the development and implementation of strategies for prevention and with the quality of life of people with the problem in question.

Target 1 – Equity in health

By the year 2000, the differences in health status between countries and between groups within countries should be reduced by at least 25%, by improving the level of health of disadvantaged nations and groups.

This target can be achieved if:

- *monitoring of differences in health status between different geographical areas and socioeconomic groups within each country is strengthened;*

- *priority is given to implementation of measures to reduce differences in health status;*

- *the basic prerequisites for health, such as food, housing and education, are available to all;*

- *living and working environments that support health are more accessible;*

- *adequate health care is made accessible to all;*

- *disadvantaged nations obtain special assistance and attention.*

Problem statement   The most widely available indicators of differences in health status in the European Region are based on mortality. Around 1980, infant mortality in different countries ranged from 91 to under 7 deaths per 1000 live births, while life expectancy at birth varied from 63 to 77 years. While there has been progress in some areas, such as infant mortality, other indicators of health status show that inequalities have continued to grow rather than decline in recent years.[a]

The main contributors to inequalities in health status are exposure to unhealthy, stressful living and working conditions, inadequate access to health and other public services, and health-damaging behaviour where the degree of choice available to the individual is restricted. These factors are often out of the direct control of the people involved and tend to cluster and reinforce each other.

Within countries, marked inequalities in health status exist between the more and the less privileged groups. Differences between socioeconomic groups are often very large and may amount to several years in life expectancy. Several studies *(3 – 13)* have shown a more than twofold difference in infant

---

[a] The information on health status presented throughout Chapter 3 is derived from a combination of Regional Office sources: two reports *(1,2)* and the health for all database.

mortality and in mortality from injuries, poisoning, violence, lung cancer and myocardial infarction, as well as a threefold difference for cirrhosis of the liver. Variations in morbidity and disability are similar to those for life expectancy. For example, a study in one Member State *(14)* has shown that 42% of people with lower incomes suffer chronic illness as opposed to 18% of the high-income group. Information on changes over time in the differences in health status between population groups is rarely available. In general, however, such differences more often appear to increase or persist than to decrease.

These major inequalities remain, despite policies in all Member States that support equity and aim to reduce inequalities in health status. There are few examples of comprehensive efforts to examine the health impact of public policy systematically among different groups and regions.

Suggested solutions   The reduction of inequalities in health status between groups and regions requires information on their real extent and on contributing factors. This would gain political recognition of the problem and ensure that priority is attached to it. Economic and social policies need to address the underlying factors.

Experience in countries shows that equity policies are implemented more effectively when decision-making is devolved to local levels and mechanisms exist for public participation at all stages.

The health sector should advocate policies that aim to improve the living and working conditions of disadvantaged people, so that their physical and social environments approach those of more fortunate groups *(15)*. This implies aiming for adequate

disposable income, adequate and safe housing, appropriate food, equal opportunities for education, high standards of occupational health and safety, and clean water supplies for the entire population. It also requires effective intersectoral action in education, housing, urban planning, agriculture and environmental protection, based on a systematic assessment of health impact in governmental and nongovernmental sectors *(16)*. Arrangements to encourage intersectoral action are needed at the international, national, federal, regional and local levels.

Policies should also aim to help people to adopt healthy lifestyles. This, too, requires intersectoral action to ensure that leisure and exercise facilities are accessible and reasonably priced, that educational facilities and programmes are universally accessible and provide information to support healthy choices, and that food distribution networks ensure wide access to inexpensive and nutritious food.

Reduction of inequalities in health status also requires equal access to health care and an uptake of services that relates to need. The geographic distribution of health care resources should reflect the needs of the entire population. Provision of high technology services for sections of the population should not be at the expense of the provision of more basic services for all. Service use should not be restricted by social or economic disadvantage, and services should be sensitive to the needs of minority groups. To achieve this, disadvantaged groups within the population will require special assistance and attention.

The effective planning and implementation of measures to reduce inequalities in health will require stronger efforts in research, monitoring and evaluation.

Many statistical systems in the health sector do not record the information needed to address the issues of equity and cannot support the monitoring and evaluation of policy and practice.

The transboundary nature of many factors contributing to inequalities in health status means that cooperation at the international level is essential. This is obvious in areas such as the control of air and water pollution. Intercountry collaboration is also important where specific assistance is offered, either directly from country to country or through WHO coordination. Turkey has, for a long time, received a particularly high proportion of the country programme budget in the European Region.

More recently, the Regional Committee, in September 1990, approved the EUROHEALTH programme to provide assistance to countries in central and eastern Europe over the next five years. This initiative demonstrates that international solidarity can be called on to deal with inequalities between countries.

While tackling this target within the European Region, the wider global context must not be neglected. The current financial crises in many developing countries in other WHO regions underlines the need for Member States in the European Region to be certain that policies aimed at improving health in their own countries do not contribute to deterioration in developing countries.

Target 2 – Health and quality of life

By the year 2000, all people should have the opportunity to develop and use their own health potential in order to lead socially, economically and mentally fulfilling lives.

This target can be achieved if:

- *monitoring of health potential and quality of life is strengthened;*

- *active participation in community life is encouraged;*

- *access to the prerequisites for health, especially education, is improved;*

- *healthy lifestyles based on effective coping skills become widely accepted;*

- *health and environmental aspects of living and working are improved and social networks strengthened;*

- *greater emphasis is placed on the quality of life in providing primary, secondary and tertiary care.*

Problem statement   Health is created and lived by people in all the settings of their everyday lives. WHO views health as a positive condition involving the whole person. It defines health as a state of complete physical, mental and social wellbeing, and not merely the absence of disease or disability. Health for all is concerned with creating structures and mechanisms that empower and support individuals in developing and using their own capabilities to the fullest extent possible. It aims to enable them to realize their full potential for health and thereby enhance the quality of their lives.

The achievement of this aim is hampered by lack of access to the prerequisites for health, especially education, by obstacles in the physical and social environment that interfere with the choice of healthy ways of living, and by health-threatening aspects of living and working environments *(17)*. The rapid social, economic and political changes that are now occurring in the European Region present new challenges to Member States to provide conditions that are supportive of health. By emphasizing a positive concept of health and an intersectoral approach to health action, these challenges can be met.

Some population groups are particularly vulnerable. They lack opportunities to use their capabilities to the full, so that they cannot develop their health potential. In some cases this creates handicaps or functional limitation. Groups particularly affected include elderly people, single parents with young children, shift or night workers, ethnic minority groups and migrant workers *(18)*, people with disabilities, people in institutions, and those living with chronic disease *(19,20)*. The particular obstacles that these groups face in developing and using their health potential need to be addressed by actions specifically tailored for them.

Suggested solutions   The achievement of this target will require policies and programmes that reflect a balanced concern with the quality of life and the physical, mental and social aspects of health.

Improvements in living and working conditions   Improvements in living and working conditions can be achieved by protecting the quality of the natural environment and by ensuring that communities have safe and adequate housing, parks and recreational areas. Both social and physical environments are important in maintaining health. A growing body of knowledge points to the health gains achieved by avoiding stress and participating actively in social networks involving families, friends and the community *(21)*. Health for all programmes need to emphasize the health benefits of social support and to strengthen the settings in which these can be achieved.

Educational programmes that aim to empower people to develop their own physical, mental and emotional capabilities play an important part in achieving this target. Preschool, school and adult education programmes should aim to improve individuals' skills in areas such as decision-making, interpersonal relationships, and coping strategies. They should help people to inform themselves about healthy lifestyles and harmful behaviour and empower them to make healthy choices.

Specific action   Certain population groups require action specifically tailored for them to help them realize their health potential and attain a good quality of life. Reallocation of resources both within and outside the health sector will be necessary to achieve this. Issues affecting specific groups are discussed further under the targets for people with disabilities (target 3), elderly people (target 6), children and young people (target 7), women (target 8), people at work (target 25) and people with special needs (target 30).

Quality of life   Quality of life is also an important issue throughout the health care system, and requires a significant adjustment of priorities and reallocation of resources. It is particularly important that care and resources are not used only to cure disease or to prolong life. Proper provision must also be made to enhance the quality of life for chronically disabled or ill people and for those who are terminally ill, who should be ensured a dignified death *(22)*.

A great deal of effort has been expended on devising means to measure the quality of life, and several instruments are now available *(23 – 28)*. Greater emphasis needs to be given to monitoring health potential and quality of life, through the use of appropriate population surveys and special studies where necessary. Monitoring many of the targets in this chapter requires quality of life measures that can be applied to disadvantaged groups to assess the extent to which they achieve equity. These groups include people with disabilities (target 3), people with chronic diseases *(29)* (targets 4, 9 and 10), elderly people *(30)* (target 6), and people with mental disorders (target 12). In some areas, suitable measurement instruments will require further development.

Target 3 – Better opportunities for people with disabilities

By the year 2000, people with disabilities should be able to lead socially, economically and mentally fulfilling lives with the support of special arrangements that improve their relative physical, social and economic opportunities.

This target aims at:

- *the provision of equal opportunities;*

- *an improvement in the status of people with disabilities;*

- *allowing people with disability to improve their quality of life and develop their health potential.*[a]

---

[a] The question of preventing the incidence of disability is closely related to many other targets, in particular targets 4, 11 and 12.

It can be achieved by implementing strategies that:

- *promote positive attitudes in society towards people with disabilities;*

- *create non-handicapping environments;*

- *promote independent living for people with disabilities, through rehabilitation and social support;*

- *provide appropriate services and support to those who do not have the functional ability to remain independent and to their families or other carers.*

Problem statement While estimates vary, about 10% of the population in the European Region probably suffers from significant long-term disability. This means that some 85 million people would benefit from policies and services to alleviate the consequences of impairment and disability. These numbers will increase as the population grows older. The main causes of disability are locomotor disorders, sight and hearing problems, injuries, mental disorders and cardiovascular disease.

There will always be people who suffer impairment and disability despite the best preventive and rehabilitative efforts, but this need not result in handicap. People with disabilities are socially handicapped when they are denied the opportunities generally available to others to enjoy family life, education, employment, housing, access to public facilities and freedom of movement. They can be helped to lead satisfying and productive lives through improvements in physical and social environments.

Despite improvements in recent years, in most European countries the integration of people with disabilities into their communities is far from satisfactory. They still suffer restricted educational opportunities because of limited mobility or because their abilities and potential are not recognized. They are often denied employment, or are given menial and poorly paid jobs, when proper training and placement could enable them to meet prevailing work standards. Children with disabilities may be confined to institutions that are more custodial than educational. People with disabilities are often denied the right to self-determination in their own lives and are unable to participate in the active life of their community. This socially inflicted deprivation is especially acute for people with mental disabilities.

To alleviate social handicap, stronger legislation is required in areas such as access to employment, transport, public services and buildings. The concept of equalizing the opportunities for independent living has not been widely adopted in the European Region and community-oriented rehabilitation is limited. The effectiveness of disability policies is often weakened by a disproportionate allocation of available resources into highly specialized technology and services for acute life-threatening conditions. The problems of impairment and disability have not been adequately addressed and intersectoral support services (health, social services, education, employment, housing) have not been coordinated. Finally, a lack of internationally comparable data on the causes and prevalence of disability and handicap has contributed to an underestimation of the extent of the problem and its economic and social impact.

Suggested solutions   All legislation and policy development should take into account, explicitly, the needs of people with disabilities *(31)*. Countries would benefit from a comprehensive policy to create equal opportunities for people with disabilities, which aims to integrate them fully into the social and economic life of their communities. Such policies need to be supported by a strategy for implementation that combines national or federal support with local action.

Health authorities should take the lead in establishing coordinated intersectoral action on behalf of people with disabilities, as well as providing effective primary care and rehabilitation services, which should be holistic, multidisciplinary, flexible and based on best current practice. Services should be delivered through community-based workers and facilities and coordinated with social welfare, education and training. Technical aids and equipment that enable people to function independently should be more readily available to people with disabilities. Some countries use institutes of technology, others rely on industry to market aids and equipment. Priority should also be given to the provision of social support for independent living. Some people will always be unable to live independently; appropriate services and

support must also be made available to them and their carers.

The successful implementation of policies to relieve handicap requires a clear definition of responsibilities for planning and monitoring, effective coordination between decision-makers and service providers, and the involvement of people with disabilities in decisions affecting them. Support is needed for the establishment or strengthening of nongovernmental organizations of people with disabilities.

Intersectoral coordination is essential for vocational training and placement, basic education, access to transport and public facilities, programmes to support independent living and the creation of non-handicapping environments. While integration within the workforce is desirable, sheltered employment for people with disabilities will be essential in some cases. In many countries, the valuable experience of local voluntary organizations can form the focus for work in this area, which may require support through legislation or regulations.

Efforts to improve opportunities for disabled people will be assisted by better comparative information about the incidence and prevalence of disability among Member States, about the aids and services that have been shown to improve physical and social independence, and about training in disability management.

Finally, positive attitudes need to be developed towards people with disabilities. This will require extensive campaigns, aimed at all age groups, to help them recognize the abilities of disabled people, and to work towards a fully integrated society.

Target 4 – Reducing chronic disease

By the year 2000 there should be a sustained and continuing reduction in morbidity and disability due to chronic disease in the Region.

This target can be achieved through:

- *a reduction of at least 10% in morbidity and disability due to chronic disease;*

- *a reduction of at least one third in diabetes complications, and particularly blindness, renal failure, amputations, pregnancy complications and coronary heart disease;*

- *a reduction in the severity of dental caries and periodontal disease to the point where children have no more than two decayed, missing or filled teeth by the age of 12 years;*

- *a sustained and continuing reduction in morbidity, disability and suffering associated with degenerative, rheumatic, neurological and chronic respiratory disease and allergies;*

- *ensuring access to genetic counselling and appropriate preventive measures for all at risk;*

- *adopting a strategy for the reduction of chronic and noncommunicable diseases (see also targets 9, 10 and 12) operating on common risk factors and integrating interventions in different sectors of the community;*

- *improving the statistical base for monitoring chronic disease, giving priority to data on years of life free from disability and major disease.*

Problem statement   This target addresses chronic diseases that are major public health problems because of the pain, suffering, inconvenience and loss of physical capacity that they cause. Increased life expectancy, together with the ability of medical technology to postpone death without always restoring health, means that the prevalence of some of these chronic conditions is increasing. The historic focus on mortality as an indicator of health policy achievement has resulted in non-life-threatening diseases receiving a relatively low priority until now. The prevention of these conditions and the alleviation of their consequences is a major challenge for health care systems. The specific cases of cardiovascular disease and cancer are considered under targets 9 and 10. The main focus of target 4 is chronic disease such as degenerative rheumatic, neurological and chronic respiratory diseases, diabetes, and allergies.

Comprehensive data on the prevalence of chronic diseases and their effects on quality of life are extremely limited. Prevalence figures for cardiovascular diseases range from 10% to 40% in different Member States, and musculoskeletal diseases from 7% to 24%. Prevalence rates are higher among older people and among those with lower socio-economic status. The consequences of noncommunicable diseases are a considerable burden to sufferers, in some cases resulting in functional impairment and handicap, and adversely affecting the quality of life over much of the life span.

Diabetes   Diabetes is a potentially life-threatening disease that remains undiagnosed in a large proportion of the population. It is estimated to affect 30 million people in the European Region. It is particularly important because of its complications, which include cardiovascular disease, blindness, renal failure, amputations and problems in pregnancy. Many of these are preventable, but effective action requires collaboration between health professionals, the community and affected individuals.

Dental disease   Recently, the frequency and severity of dental caries and periodontal disease have fallen dramatically in a number of countries, though in others the rates are unchanged or increasing. The global goal of no more than three decayed, missing or filled teeth at the age of 12 years has already been achieved in 53% of the relevant population in the Region.

Allergy   Basic knowledge about hypersensitivity and allergic conditions has advanced in recent years. Information on the prevalence and consequences of allergies is still inadequate, though possible recent increases have been attributed to changes in lifestyle and eating habits. Recent findings show that food allergies can be much more frequent, and with more varied symptomatology, than previously recognized. There is also concern about smoking as a co-factor in allergies.

Genetically determined conditions   Genetically determined conditions, such as thalassaemia major and neural tube defects, which cause major disability, impairment and discomfort, are receiving increasing attention in the Region because of a greater understanding of their extent and better opportunities for early detection, prevention and treatment.

Suggested solutions   Progress towards this target will be affected by action on cardiovascular disease (target 9), cancer (target 10), accidents (target 11), mental disorders (target 12) and the health of people at work (target 25).

Policy development   People in the Region would benefit from comprehensive policies on the prevention of chronic noncommunicable diseases and the alleviation of their consequences. A useful approach is the countrywide integrated noncommunicable disease intervention (CINDI) programme *(32,33)*, which emphasizes primary care, multisectoral action and community participation. Each policy needs to take account of the specific characteristics of the particular disease and must encourage close collaboration with community groups, especially those that represent people suffering from chronic conditions.

Service provision   Service provision should be coordinated intersectorally, building on cooperative action with all other relevant agencies, such as social services, and fitness and recreation services. It should actively support the partners, families and friends involved in the care of individuals with chronic disease. Some countries already have policies that provide a framework for the development of networks of community care and social support centres for people with particular chronic diseases. Practical measures that can be taken to alleviate the pain and loss of function associated with chronic diseases include specific therapeutic measures such as joint replacement, physical fitness training, dietary change, lifestyle adjustment and rehabilitation services. Technical aids that can enhance the functional capacity for independent living should be developed and made readily available.

Environmental improvement   General environmental measures such as pollution control will make an important contribution to the alleviation of the consequences of respiratory disease. Specific moves to control tobacco consumption, through the control of smoking in public and support for smoking prevention and cessation, are also important in reducing the consequences of these conditions *(34)*.

Diabetes   A diabetes strategy should focus on the early identification and management of the disease based on an active partnership between health professionals and diabetic individuals. Major initiatives to improve diabetes care and reduce its complications have been taken by health departments in Member States in cooperation with the International Diabetes Federation and WHO, resulting in the St Vincent Declaration in October 1989 *(35)*. The development of baseline data for the monitoring of diabetes complications is a priority for the years ahead.

Dental disease   Primary prevention strategies require the education of children, parents and teachers. Fluoridation of drinking-water has a role to play. It remains controversial in some regions and localities, where alternative preventive approaches such as the use of fluoride salt, toothpastes, gels or tablets should be developed. Other important measures are incentives for dentists to prevent secondary caries.

Asthma   The effective recognition and treatment of asthma offers the scope to reduce associated mortality and morbidity. Therapy can be directed at the prevention of attacks and the early recognition and effective treatment of attacks, which will minimize side-effects and treatment-induced complications. Peak flow meters can enable individuals to measure their own lung function and thus contribute to early intervention.

Allergies   Further research is required to establish the underlying etiology of most allergies. Until this is achieved, guidelines for the design of intervention programmes cannot be drawn up. Where prevention is not possible, emphasis should be placed on improving treatment regimes to reduce associated morbidity, and on reducing exposure to suspected co-factors, such as smoking. A reduction in the chemicals in food and in the environment may also have a positive impact.

Genetically determined conditions   Progress in this area will require greater public awareness of the conditions involved and their causes. Action is required to promote ready access to genetic counselling, fetal diagnosis and related services. This may involve screening during childhood, before conception, early in pregnancy and in the neonatal period *(36)*. In some countries, the use of prenatal screening services has resulted in the reduced incidence, or even elimination, of certain genetically determined conditions. The extremely important and difficult ethical issues involved make it essential that technical interventions are used only when the individuals concerned are offered an extensive, informed choice.

Information   To measure progress towards this target, action needs to be taken to improve the statistical base for monitoring chronic disease and its effects. Priority should be given to monitoring life spans free of disability. Such data are currently available in only a few Member States. Measuring the quality of life for people with chronic disease is also important. Priorities for the future also include new approaches to research, to determine the incidence and prevalence of these diseases and their associated consequences, and training geared to primary care and community support.

Target 5 – Reducing communicable disease

By the year 2000, there should be no indigenous cases of poliomyelitis, diphtheria, neonatal tetanus, measles, mumps and congenital rubella in the Region and there should be a sustained and continuing reduction in the incidence and adverse consequences of other communicable diseases, notably HIV infection.

This target can be achieved by control strategies implemented through well organized health care systems ensuring effective epidemiological surveillance, education, treatment and care and aimed at achieving:

- *vaccination of all eligible people against eradicable diseases and other communicable diseases that can be contained with vaccination;*

- *a sustained and continuing reduction in the rate of transmission of HIV infection and alleviation of its negative consequences, including social reactions to people with HIV infection and AIDS;*

- *a reduction of 25% in the mortality associated with pneumonia and diarrhoeal diseases in children and with hepatitis B;*

- *a sustained and continuing reduction in the rate of transmission of, and severe complications associated with, sexually transmitted diseases.*

Problem statement Communicable disease in the European Region remains an important cause of morbidity. Almost one third of the population is affected by communicable disease or its associated complications each year *(37)*.

Diseases controlled by vaccination The elimination of measles requires immunization coverage close to 100%, but in 1989/1990 some 30% of the total population of the Region lived in countries where immunization rates were below 80%. A drastic change in attitudes towards vaccination will be needed to eliminate measles throughout the Region by the year 2000. Mumps and rubella can be eliminated with lower immunization rates than for measles *(38,39)*.

HIV infection and AIDS Infection with the human immunodeficiency virus (HIV) remains a serious challenge because of its consequences, the lack of effective treatment and the present limited opportunities for prevention. Some 48 000 cases of acquired immunodeficiency syndrome (AIDS) had been reported in the Region by early 1991. About 500 000 Europeans were estimated to have contracted HIV infection by the end of 1990 *(40)*. This total could reach 1.5 million by the year 2000, when heterosexual transmission may be the primary mode of transmission. The chronic nature of AIDS, which can last for months or years, and the need for medical, nursing, counselling and social services is placing new pressures on the organization and financing of health services. The social stigma and discrimination associated with the disease is raising special problems in terms of violation of individual rights and loss of social support for people who are HIV positive.

Other diseases not controlled by vaccination Other diseases such as acute respiratory infections,

including pneumonia, and diarrhoeal disease can also be largely controlled through better case management, especially in children and infants *(41)*.

Suggested solutions Several diseases can be eliminated if effective measures are taken, and the incidence and consequences of others can be substantially reduced.

Diseases controlled by vaccination Strategies for the control of communicable diseases that are preventable through immunization have been developed under the auspices of WHO and are incorporated in the Expanded Programme on Immunization (EPI). Country programmes, based on these strategies, have achieved remarkable progress. They aim to increase immunization coverage, improve surveillance at the regional, national, federal and local levels, develop laboratory services and ensure vaccine quality. The development of a combined vaccine for measles, mumps and rubella allows a common approach to these diseases, and experience in some Member States indicates that eradication of these diseases is possible. These technical programmes have to be accompanied by training for health personnel and encouragement of community action if they are to be fully effective.

HIV infection and AIDS A reduction in the rate of HIV transmission can at present only be achieved through energetic health education and health promotion programmes that are integrated with public health and treatment services. An effective strategy involves striking a balance. It needs to be based on an epidemiological assessment that includes the use of diagnostic facilities, seroepidemiological surveys and seroprevalence data reporting. It must include health promotion, particularly information and education to encourage safer sexual practices among the general population as well as among individuals who practise high-risk behaviour. Preventing the spread of infection through blood supplies requires a safe supply of blood, the correct use of blood and blood products, and the screening of blood and organ donors. The prevention of perinatal transmission requires intensive and widespread health education and outreach, aimed particularly at injecting drug users and their sexual partners. All these approaches to the prevention of HIV transmission have to be sensitive to the social, cultural and linguistic characteristics of the population and carried out in close cooperation with nongovernmental organizations working in the field.

When developing programmes for diagnosis, counselling, care and clinical management, existing facilities and personnel need to be assessed to determine where increases in or reallocation of resources are required to ensure that coordinated and comprehensive services can be provided. The psychological and social effects of HIV infection and AIDS mean that information, education and counselling must be available to those affected by the disease, their partners and others with whom they have contact *(42)*. Measures are also needed to ensure that the basic human rights of those suffering from HIV infection are protected and to change the negative societal attitudes underlying discrimination and other adverse social reactions towards people who are HIV positive or who have AIDS. Finally, the evaluation of health promotion work

on HIV infection and AIDS is an important priority, together with the dissemination of results both within and between countries.

Other diseases not controlled by vaccination
Mortality associated with diarrhoeal disease in children can be reduced through higher hygiene standards, the provision of safe drinking-water and food, the use of oral rehydration salt and the prompt delivery of other appropriate medical care at the primary level. The reduction of mortality associated with pneumonia in children requires improvements in case management and effective access to medical care services to facilitate early diagnosis.

More effective targeting of at-risk populations will serve to decrease the incidence of acute hepatitis B. In the long term, effective vaccination policies will be associated with a decrease in the carrier state and hence a reduction in mortality associated with chronic disease. In the short term, mortality associated with chronic disease may be reduced slightly through better management of chronic liver disease and treatment with interferon.

The rate of transmission of major sexually transmitted diseases can be reduced and severe complications prevented by systematic health education for prevention backed up by early diagnosis and treatment, carried out within a well organized primary health care system.

Target 6 – Healthy aging

By the year 2000, life expectancy at birth in the Region should be at least 75 years and there should be a sustained and continuing improvement in the health of all people aged 65 years and over.

This target aims at achieving:

- *an increase in life expectancy at birth to at least 67 years for men and 74 years for women in every country in the Region;*[a]

- *a reduction of at least 25% in the differences in life expectancy at birth among geographical areas and socioeconomic groups and between the sexes;*

- *an increase in the number of years people aged 65 and over live free from disability, and an improvement in the quality of their lives.*

It can be achieved by implementing strategies that:

- *encourage full and active participation of the elderly in community life;*

- *prolong the period of healthy aging through lifestyle changes and supportive environments;*

- *provide appropriate services and support to elderly people in need.*

[a] These figures refer to life expectancy in individual countries, whereas the figure of 75 years in the target itself relates to life expectancy in the Region as a whole.

Problem statement   Life expectancy at birth varies throughout the Region, both between countries and between groups within countries. The most recent figures available, for around 1989/1990, range from 74 to 64 years for men across the different countries in the Region and from 81 to 69 years for women; 47% of the total population of the Region live in countries where male life expectancy at birth is under 67 years, but only 16% of the total regional population live in countries where female life expectancy is less than 74 years. The achievement of an overall life expectancy of 75 years for the Region as a whole by the year 2000 depends particularly on progress in the central, eastern and southern parts of the Region.

In 1960, 14.4% of the European population were over the age of 60 years. By 1980, this proportion had increased to 16.9% and it will rise to 20.2% by the year 2000. The age group that is growing most rapidly is the over 80s. The number of people in this age group is predicted to grow from 16 million to 21 million between 1980 and 2000. These demographic changes will have profound implications for the future of health policy and health services, especially long-term care. If the needs of the elderly are to be met effectively within the boundaries of sustainable cost, policies and programmes will have to be adopted that help the elderly to remain active and healthy for as long as possible.

Improvements in care and the increased survival of the sick have led to a shift in emphasis from prolonging life expectancy to increasing the expectation of active life or of life free of disability. Although reduced functional capacity is correlated with advancing age, what percentage of reduced function is due to preventable loss of fitness and/or social contacts is not clear. Many aging people do not show symptoms of mental or physical decline; on the contrary, they tend to enjoy a level of health that permits them to lead socially and economically healthy lives. Seven out of ten people in the age group 70–80 years require no assistance in caring for themselves *(43)*.

Morbidity in the aged is characterized by multiple pathology, nonspecific presentation and a high incidence of complications of both disease and treatment. About 20% of those aged 60 or older are free of symptoms *(44)*. Of the remainder, a large proportion report more than one condition or symptom. The most common problems are arthritis, reduced vision and hearing, dementia, depression, sleep disturbance, incontinence, unsteadiness, social isolation and institutionalization. These problems must receive priority in action and research to achieve healthy aging.

During this century, the average educational level and socioeconomic conditions of the elderly have improved. These changes contribute to better health status and also mean that in the future the elderly will be better informed, more politically involved and able to participate more actively in community life. New problems are emerging, however, because of the migration of younger generations, the entry of more women into the workforce and the greater complexity of everyday life. These changes lead to more social isolation among the elderly and fewer informal carers to support them. Other formal care arrangements therefore have to be planned.

Aging and health tend to be low priorities in the government policies of most Member States. Health promotion and disease prevention programmes geared to the needs of older people are poorly developed in such areas as physical activity, appropriate eating, reduction of alcohol use, control of prescription drugs and maintenance of social networks and security. Most areas have few community structures for care and social support, and more effort is needed to improve the accessibility of housing, transport and community activity.

Suggested solutions   Each country needs a comprehensive policy to create better opportunities for healthy aging, based on the objective of maintaining maximum functional capacity throughout the latter years of life and balancing this with appropriate care where needed. The policy needs to be supported by a strategy for implementation that combines national or federal support with local action. The health sector should act as a strong advocate for comprehensive economic and social policies that enhance the relative position of the elderly. Health authorities can also act as advocates for coordinated intersectoral action on behalf of the elderly while providing effective primary care, rehabilitative services and institutional facilities where needed.

The successful implementation of policies to make the latter years of life as healthy as possible requires a clear delineation of the responsibilities for planning and monitoring it, effective coordination between relevant decision-makers and service providers, and the involvement of elderly people in decisions affecting them. Appropriate mechanisms to achieve this will vary according to circumstances. National, federal, regional or local bodies may be assigned special responsibility for the elderly. To be effective, such bodies require ready access to decision-makers and representation from the elderly.

Broad central policies should provide the framework within which coordinated local action, involving governmental and nongovernmental organizations, can be taken to address key areas. These include income support, retirement practices, housing and transport, catering services, fitness and recreational activities, and opportunities for participation in community life. The prevention of social isolation has been shown to help maintain functional capacity and support healthy aging. It can be achieved by measures such as providing better educational opportunities for those aged over 65, for example through universities of the third age, and creating specific organizations that allow older people to use their knowledge and experience for the benefit of the whole community. One Member State has done this by setting up town councils of the wise.

Efforts need to be focused on maintaining physical fitness for as long as possible. This presupposes educating people in healthy lifestyles, in the management of stress, in the need for adequate exercise and nutrition, and in the prevention of loss of autonomy as well as the prevention of disease. This process should begin in middle age to be fully effective, although many benefits can still be gained from lifestyle changes late in life.

More intensive efforts should be made to spread current knowledge about the aging process and ways of maintaining functional capacity and postponing the onset of chronic disease and disability. Training and research towards this end should receive higher priority.

The future rapid growth in numbers of people aged 85 years and over will create a special demand for new programmes and facilities to provide long-term care. These will need to achieve a balance between institutional care and community services, with a high degree of coordination between health, social services and the voluntary sector. Providing information and effective means of support for self-help groups and informal care givers is also particularly important. This support will need to be strengthened and supplemented in future when the proportion of people in the middle age groups, from which many informal care givers are drawn, falls. It will be a particular challenge to provide humane, high quality care within the bounds of acceptable cost.

A specific policy goal should be to provide opportunities and encouragement for those aged over 65 to remain active participants in the social and cultural life of the communities to which they belong. They should be regarded not as a burden, or as medical and social problems, but as a valuable resource, bringing life experience and wisdom to their communities.

Target 7 – Health of children and young people

By the year 2000, the health of all children and young people should be improved, giving them the opportunity to grow and develop to their full physical, mental and social potential.

This target aims at achieving:

- *comprehensive support of children and their families, according to their health needs and socioeconomic circumstances;*

- *a reduction of infant mortality rates in countries with rates currently between 10 and 20 per 1000 live births to below 10, and in countries with rates currently above 20 per 1000 live births to below 15;*

- *a reduction of 25% in the differences in infant mortality rates between geographical areas and socioeconomic groups;*

- *a reduction of 25% in mortality and serious injury in children and young people, notably due to accidents.*

It can be achieved by implementing strategies that:

- *protect children as vulnerable members of society, with all appropriate measures in accordance with the United Nations Convention on the Rights of the Child;*

- *organize disease prevention and health surveillance for all children, including good antenatal, postnatal, preschool and school health services;*

- *promote breastfeeding of infants by the greatest possible proportion of mothers, including working mothers;*

- *promote healthy patterns of living among children and young people;*

- *ensure social, economic and psychological support for disadvantaged children, including those with long-term illness and disability, and for their families;*

- *ensure that all young people are informed about, and have easy access to, facilities and support to avoid unplanned parenthood.*

Problem statement   There are several major reasons why the health and wellbeing of children and young people are of special importance in a country's health policy. They make up a substantial part of each country's population, on average around 20% in the Region as a whole. Improving the health of young people and their attitudes to health behaviour is an important humanitarian and economic investment. They are a vulnerable group in society, often lacking political power, and their health and wellbeing thus reflect the will and ability of society to care for all its citizens. This vulnerability is perhaps most clearly seen in the problem of child abuse, including sexual abuse, which is a significant problem in all sections of society. Adult knowledge, attitudes and behaviour in health matters are learned and cemented in the formative years of childhood and youth. The United Nations has proposed special protection for children through its Convention on the Rights of the

Child, adopted in 1989, which applies to all those aged under 18 years unless national or federal laws recognize an earlier age of majority *(45)*.

Childhood mortality   In most countries of the Region, childhood mortality has now reached a comparatively low level. Efforts are still required, however, to decrease mortality differences between countries and between socioeconomic, ethnic and other subgroups within countries. Infant mortality rates have continued to decline in recent years in countries throughout the Region. Nevertheless, according to the latest available data from around 1989, 20% of the total population of the Region live in countries where rates are above 20 per 1000 live births. For these countries, action is still required to continue the reduction in the infant mortality rate. The problem of sudden infant death syndrome (SIDS) must also be tackled, which is estimated to account for 1.5 to 2.5 infant deaths per 1000 live births *(46)*. Accidents, especially road accidents, are particularly important as a cause of mortality and disability, being the cause of about one quarter of all deaths in children aged 5 – 14 years and one third in young people aged 15 – 24 years.

Childhood morbidity   Greater medical knowledge and better technology mean that more children survive premature birth, congenital malformations, accidents and malignant diseases. Their survival is often not free of disability and handicap. This, in conjunction with the growing prevalence of environmentally provoked diseases such as allergies, means that long-term health problems will increase among children and young people. They and their families require comprehensive, continuous and coordinated social, psychological and economic support. These developments raise ethical

issues and questions of priority that have hitherto not needed to be addressed.

In many parts of the Region, infections and other traditional threats to children's health have declined in importance, but vigilance is still needed. The maintenance of the established health protection and disease prevention programmes, especially immunization, is of prime importance.

Some children are more exposed to the risk of ill health than others: children in and after wars, refugees, immigrants, children from ethnic minorities, and children from poor families. Their specific problems may include mental health problems *(18)*, anxiety, problems with relationships, and aggressive behaviour. All of these may have further consequences in their adult lives.

Although the consequences of substance abuse (alcohol, tobacco and illicit drugs) will usually appear as physical, mental and social injuries in adulthood, increasingly the abusive behaviour is established in childhood and adolescence. A recent survey *(47)* in the European Community among young people aged 11 – 15 years showed that 61% have already had contact with alcohol, and 14% could be considered regular drinkers (i.e. they drink wine, beer, apéritifs or spirits at least once a week). Data on smoking from the same survey showed that, in 1990, 5% of the 11 – 15 year olds already smoked at least once a week. An earlier study *(48)* in 11 European countries revealed that by the age of 15, only one third of children reported they had never smoked.

Suggested solutions   Better health for children and young people can be attained only by multisectoral efforts. The first step is to ensure politically that their rights as human beings and members of society are protected according to the United Nations Convention *(45)*. The Convention treats the civil, political, economic, social and cultural rights of children as elements in an interdependent, mutually reinforcing package. It emphasizes the right of every child to participate in decisions affecting both the present and the future. The empowerment of children to exercise this and other rights can be facilitated through education and other means that support the development of self esteem, skills and abilities. The Convention specifically mentions the rights of all children to the highest standard of health and medical care available, and to protection from abuse, neglect and other threats to health and wellbeing.

Policy development   Countries will benefit from a comprehensive policy that aims to protect the health of children and young people and to promote the development of healthy patterns of living. An important component will be strategies to prevent the abuse of children and young people, for example through violence, sexual abuse (including child prostitution) and economic exploitation.

Health goals already achieved should be continuously defended by programmes of prevention, health surveillance, family support, care and rehabilitation. Important components include good antenatal and postnatal care as well as preschool and school health services. All young people should have the necessary information and access to services, counselling and other support to prevent unplanned parenthood. Although all these programmes should be directed towards the whole population of children and families, special attention should be paid to the least privileged groups and the individuals at greatest risk. The outcomes of these programmes need to be continuously evaluated.

Special emphasis should be put on social and economic factors as causes and consequences of ill health. One important area is the protection of children and young people from the harmful effects of others' smoking, through establishing their right to a smoke-free environment (one of the principles formulated at the Madrid conference *(34)* on action on smoking).

Breastfeeding   Continued action is necessary in some parts of the Region both to sustain reductions in the overall level of infant mortality and to reduce the differences between geographic areas and socioeconomic groups within countries. The promotion of breastfeeding by the greatest possible proportion of mothers, including working mothers, should be encouraged. Health professionals need to play a sensitive and supportive role in encouraging women to establish and continue breastfeeding. This can be supported by legislation on maternity leave, appropriate hospital ward routines and the implementation of the 1981 International Code of Marketing of Breast-milk Substitutes *(49,50)*.

Health promotion   The fact that children and young people depend to a great extent on other individuals for protection and care, and are influenced by the behavioural patterns they witness, makes them vulnerable but also offers opportunities for health promotion activities. Attitudes and behaviours developed in childhood and adolescence related to diet, exercise, sexual practices, safety habits and the use of tobacco, alcohol and psychoactive drugs have health consequences that continue throughout life. Schools are particularly important as settings in which programmes can be geared to encourage high self-esteem, interest in physical activity and the adoption of healthy lifestyles *(51,52)*.

They can provide individuals with accurate information and empower them to take their own decisions. Youth organizations, clubs and sports movements also have an important role in promoting healthy lifestyles among young people *(53)*. Actions taken in response to targets 14, 15, 16 and 17 will also be relevant here.

Long-term disability   Finally, for children and young people with long-term illness and disability, appropriate intersectoral mechanisms need to be set up to ensure that they, and their families, receive the necessary social, psychological and economic support to allow them to live to the fullest extent of their capabilities. Actions taken relating to the targets on better opportunities for people with disabilities (target 3) and on community

services to meet special needs (target 30) will also be relevant here.

Related targets   The reduction of mortality and injury due to accidents among children and young people is discussed as part of the specific target on accidents (target 11), and the reduction of mortality from pneumonia and diarrhoeal diseases in the target on communicable diseases (target 5).

Information   To deepen our knowledge as a basis for action and its evaluation, documentation on the health and wellbeing of children and young people should be improved. This should include the viewpoints of children and young people and be collected in a systematic way that suits the social context.

Target 8 – Health of women

By the year 2000, there should be sustained and continuing improvement in the health of all women.

This target aims at achieving:

- *a reduction in maternal mortality to less than 15 per 100 000 live births;*

- *a substantial reduction in health problems that are unique to women;*

- *a substantial reduction in health problems of women related to their socio-economic status and the burden of their multiple roles;*

- *a substantial reduction in the incidence and adverse health consequences of sexual harassment, domestic violence and rape;*

- *sustained support for women providing informal health care;*

- *a reduction of at least 25% in the differences in maternal mortality rates between geographical areas and socioeconomic groups.*

It can be achieved by implementing strategies that:

- *pay special attention to women's health;*

- *provide improved support and care during pregnancy, including the balanced use of perinatal technology;*

- *accordingly make significant changes in the social environment and in lifestyle patterns.*

Problem statement   Women are one of the groups in the population that often suffer relative disadvantage in terms of their health and social status. Women have unique health needs that require specific and tailored action within the health and other sectors. They have health problems connected with the reproductive function and the menopause; health problems related to women's socioeconomic status, including violence, rape and other sexual harassment and abuse; and health problems and a need for support that relate to women's multiple roles in society, especially for those women providing maternal or informal health care.

The most frequently used indicators of health status are based on mortality data, and such indicators suggest that the health of women is better than that of men. Nevertheless, the more limited data available on morbidity often indicate higher levels in women than in men. In terms of self-reported levels of health, in 11 out of the 12 Member States where this information is available, a lower percentage of women than men reported their health as fair/average or better than average. The differences in reported health between women and men seem to be greater in those populations with poorer health.

These indicators, however, do not adequately describe the particular health problems that women experience. Women tend to see their health in a social context, and not just in terms of illness or injury. Dissatisfaction with a purely physical approach to health and ill health has led in all countries of the Region to the establishment of women's self-help groups. These groups focus on a wide array of issues, using a range of methods to try to put women's health affairs on public and political agendas.

The unique health problems of women are related primarily to the reproductive function. The most important of these are breast and cervical cancer (covered under target 10), genitourinary infections and pelvic inflammatory disease. Sexually transmitted diseases, notably chlamydia, also pose a widespread, though often unrecognized, threat to women's health and fertility. Comprehensive data on the prevalence and consequences of pelvic inflammatory disease are not available throughout the Region. The scale of the problem can be illustrated, however, by figures from studies elsewhere. They estimate that the risk of pelvic inflammatory disease in women aged 15 – 19 years is 1 in 8 *(54)*, and that pelvic inflammatory disease accounts for up to 20% of hospital admissions for gynaeco-logical problems and is associated with health care costs in the United States of over one billion dollars annually *(55)*.

Although maternal mortality is no longer a major problem in most countries in the Region, 48% of the total population of the Region still live in countries with maternal mortality rates above 15 per 100 000 live births. In most of these countries, trends appear to be decreasing, however, in some cases clearly linked to better access to facilities for fertility control. Of particular concern are those countries, covering some 1.5% of the total regional population, where maternal mortality rates in 1990 were higher than in 1980.

Women's health problems differ according to their age. The problems of young women tend to be associated with limited information and experience in dealing with everyday health issues and with securing access to appropriate health services. They tend to centre around the mental and social consequences of adolescent pregnancy, a higher incidence of sexual harassment and the consequences of low socioeconomic status. Middle-aged women experience the stress and negative consequences of fulfilling multiple roles both as workers and as providers of care for their families. Elderly women are often deprived of the opportunity to lead a productive life and encounter negative stereotyping. Health care providers tend to ignore the fact that the health of older men and women is influenced by different physical and social factors. Older women have to cope longer with chronic conditions such as osteoporosis, rheumatoid arthritis, obesity, hypertension, diabetes, and consequent mobility problems. The effects are compounded where criteria for social security, such as disability determinations, and pension benefits do not apply to men and women equally.

The relative social position of women has a significant influence on their health status. Violence, rape and other sexual harassment and abuse can affect women of all ages. Incidents may be domestic, involving family members, may occur at the workplace, involving colleagues or bosses, or may occur in public places. Evidence is now growing about the extent of these problems and their long-term effects on the health of women. The health sector alone cannot deal with these problems. Promising initiatives and specific projects have been developed in some places, often based around self-help groups that women themselves have initiated.

Women's economic situation is generally less favourable than that of men. Poverty is a general indicator for ill health but, in a survey in one Member State *(56)*, proportionally more women than men in low-income groups report their health as being less than good. In some countries, adequate child support is still lacking, causing social and economic problems for working mothers. Women often receive less formal education and are often engaged in work that pays less, is less interesting and is of relatively low status. Limited access to full reproductive choice through education, means of contraception and access to safe abortion can also diminish health status.

Suggested solutions   These suggested solutions follow the lines of a number of international conventions, agreements and decisions. Member States are urged to adopt, or implement their existing commitments to:

– the Nairobi Forward-Looking Strategies for the Advancement of Women (in particular, paragraphs 148 – 162 on health) and related

United Nations Economic and Social Council resolution E/CN.6/1990/L.25;

- the United Nations Convention on the Elimination of All Forms of Discrimination Against Women and the Convention on the Political Rights of Women;
- World Health Assembly resolution WHA38.27 on women, health and development and follow-up reports;
- United Nations General Assembly resolution 44/76 on elderly women; and
- Council of Europe recommendations on social measures concerning violence within the family (R(90)2) and on the elimination of sexism from language (R(90)4).

Policy development   Every country would benefit from a comprehensive policy to promote the health of women. This should aim to secure significant changes in the social environment and lifestyle patterns that influence the relative position of women and should address their specific health needs. The policy needs to be supported by a strategy for implementation that combines national or federal support with local action. Health authorities can act as advocates and can be role models for coordinated economic and social policies that support women's health. They can also develop primary and secondary care services that are acceptable to women and sensitive to their needs.

Intersectoral policies are needed to promote the health of women. They are most likely to be effective, however, if they are planned and monitored by a specific authority that has overall coordinating responsibility. Such a body must have access to decision-makers in key areas and include representatives of women's groups. This is in accordance with one of the recommendations made at the

Adelaide conference on healthy public policy *(57)*, which states that:

> for their effective participation in health promotion women require access to information, networks, and funds. All women, especially those from ethnic, indigenous, and minority groups, have the *right to self-determination of their health*, and should be full partners in the formulation of healthy public policy to ensure its cultural relevance.

In all countries of the Region, women's voluntary and self-help groups already play an important role in the promotion and protection of women's health. Policy on women's health should not aim to replace or institutionalize these groups. It should rather create the conditions under which women's health can be promoted. There are a few examples of such comprehensive policies, such as the National Agenda for Women, including the National Policy on Women's Health, established in 1988 in Australia *(58,59)*. The following suggestions draw on these documents, as well as on the WHO report *Positive approaches to promoting women's health (60)*.

Activities and policies to attain this target should address issues affecting women's total life span, and not just their reproductive years. These issues should include reproductive health and sexuality, aging, emotional and mental health, violence against women, occupational health and safety in professional and domestic workplaces, the multiple needs of female carers, and the health effects of sex role stereotyping.

Specific action needs to be taken in a number of areas. Services to meet women's particular health needs should be improved, including health information adequately aimed at women. They should be given satisfactory access to advice on fertility control, contraception and the safe termination of pregnancy (within constitutional and legislative constraints). Support and care during pregnancy should be improved and the use of perinatal technology should be balanced. Facilities dealing with different aspects of women's health should be integrated (such as services for sexually transmitted diseases, cancer screening and contraception). Appropriate measures should be taken to prevent and control problems due to chlamydia. Research and data collection should be promoted in all relevant areas. Women should participate in decision-making about all matters pertaining to community and personal health, including the training of providers of care, the allocation of resources, monitoring the effectiveness and quality of services, legislative and regulatory action, and consciousness-raising.

Target 9 – Reducing cardiovascular disease

By the year 2000, mortality from diseases of the circulatory system should be reduced, in the case of people under 65 years by at least 15%, and there should be progress in improving the quality of life of all people suffering from cardiovascular disease.

This target can be achieved by:

- *implementing preventive measures acceptable to the population that aim at reducing the levels of major risk factors such as smoking, hypertension, hypercholesterolaemia, overweight and a sedentary lifestyle;*

- *improving access to effective and acceptable methods of diagnosis, including early diagnosis, and treatment;*

- *providing physical, psychological and social rehabilitation for people with cardiovascular disease.*

Problem statement   Cardiovascular diseases are a major public health problem in Europe. In 1985, they caused 35% of the deaths among men and 30% of the deaths among women in the 25 – 64 year age group in the Region, while for the population aged 65 and older they accounted for 54% of all male deaths and 60% of all female deaths. These diseases account for about one third of permanent disability and a large portion of health care costs.

Cardiovascular disease mortality rates have declined significantly in the European Region. If current trends continue, countries covering 44% of the total population in the Region are likely to achieve the

15% reduction in mortality for people under 65 by the year 2000 called for in the target. The rate of decline in cardiovascular disease has accelerated since 1980. For example, the average regional mortality rate per 100 000 people under 65 has dropped by around 1.5 annually since 1980, compared with 0.5 in the previous decade. Although cardiovascular disease mortality rates increase with age, in some countries decreases have been observed for people over the age of 65 as well as for younger groups. To date, the decline among older people has been more rapid for women than for men. Increasing survival rates suggest a growing prevalence of cardiovascular disease morbidity and associated disability.

Cardiovascular disease mortality rates differ greatly between countries. Around 1988, age-standardized mortality rates for men aged under 65 years varied from a high of 256 per 100 000 population to a low of 70. The rates for women in the same age group varied between a high of 104 per 100 000 and a low of 22. For age groups over the age of 65, the variation between the countries with the highest and lowest mortality rates is three- to fourfold for men and three- to fivefold for women. The highest mortality rates occur in central and eastern Europe. These differences indicate a large untapped potential for preventive action.

During the 1980s, age-standardized rates of ischaemic heart disease declined substantially in both sexes under the age of 65, in countries in the north and west of the Region. In several countries, dramatic declines have begun to occur after several decades of rising mortality rates. In other countries, however, most of which are located in the central and eastern part of the Region, rates increased substantially during the 1980s.

The risk of cardiovascular disease is significantly influenced by a number of individual and population characteristics. The links between habitual diet, levels of blood cholesterol-lipoprotein and cardiovascular disease are well established. Smoking, especially of cigarettes, contributes significantly to coronary heart disease. High alcohol intake increases the risk of cardiovascular disease as well as high blood pressure. Lack of physical activity is associated with high levels of the other major risk factors.

Suggested solutions   The most effective way to reduce the mortality and morbidity associated with cardiovascular disease is by the promotion of healthy lifestyles. The key aims are prevention of smoking (both preventing people starting to smoke and helping smokers to stop), promotion of physical fitness, promotion of balanced nutrition including a lower intake of saturated fat and salt in the diet, and better stress management. This calls for countrywide community-based programmes supported by appropriate national or federal and local economic and social policy, in areas such as food and nutrition, tobacco, alcohol, and fitness and leisure facilities. The active participation of the community and the involvement of the mass media are essential. Several countries have adopted comprehensive approaches to cardiovascular disease prevention, including those participating in the CINDI and MONICA (on monitoring trends in cardiovascular diseases) projects. Several countries now have smoking prevention strategies and nutrition policies that are beginning to show positive results. Measures discussed under the targets on healthy living (target 16) and on dealing with smoking reduction (target 17) will also contribute to the achievement of this target.

This primary prevention strategy can be supplemented by a strategy for dealing with high-risk groups in the population, by identifying and helping individuals in need of special protection. This will include the use of both non-drug and drug treatment to control hypertension and reduce serum cholesterol levels.

For patients suffering from cardiovascular disease, the priority should be avoiding the recurrence and progression of the disease. Improved access to effective and acceptable methods of diagnosis and treatment is very important in reducing the effects of cardiovascular disease. Comprehensive care should include physical, psychological and social rehabilitation, and advice on the modification of behaviour to reduce risk. Attention also needs to be given to the quality of care and the use of

appropriate technology (further discussed under target 31). Continued research is needed into the quality and cost-effectiveness of surgical and nonsurgical treatments. The quality of life of people with cardiovascular disease must also be maintained and monitored.

Finally, priority must be assigned to this issue by making greater efforts to promote the spread of the knowledge that has been obtained and to initiate changes in the structure and practices of the health sector. This will involve a reallocation of resources, stronger emphasis on prevention in health service practice and new approaches to training primary health care workers.

Target 10 – Controlling cancer

By the year 2000, mortality from cancer in people under 65 years should be reduced by at least 15% and the quality of life of all people with cancer should be significantly improved.

This target can be achieved if:

- *the incidence of tobacco-related cancer is reduced as a result of major efforts to decrease smoking rates;*

- *cervical and breast cancer mortality is reduced through the establishment of screening and early treatment programmes including steps to improve acceptance;*

- *living and working environments are made more healthy;*

- *the best available knowledge in diagnosis, treatment, rehabilitation and palliative care is applied in an appropriate way to all people with cancer.*

Problem statement   Cancer is a major public health problem and an important concern for people in the Region. In 1985, for the European Region as a whole, cancer caused about 30% of all deaths among men and 40% of those among women in the age group 25 – 64 years. Although some countries show decreasing trends for standardized mortality from cancer in people aged under 65, nearly two thirds of the population of the Region live in countries where cancer mortality is still increasing.

Cancer mortality varies considerably between countries. Around 1988, for those aged under 65, mortality rates ranged from 175 to 67 per 100 000 population for men and from 107 to 56 for women. The countries in the central and eastern part of the Region have the highest mortality and the most unfavourable trends.

The increase in overall cancer mortality during the 1980s has been due mainly to lung cancer, which accounts for around one third of all cancer deaths in middle-aged men. Breast cancer is the leading cause of death from cancer among women in all countries. Mortality rates for breast cancer are increasing in most countries for both under and over 65-year-olds, though the rates vary considerably between countries. Mortality rates from cervical cancer are decreasing in most countries for both age groups, 0 – 64 years and 65 years and over, although they vary considerably between countries. Some countries have reported an increase in the incidence of melanoma, predominantly due to overexposure to sunlight.

The risk factors associated with cancer present a mixed picture. The prevalence of smoking has decreased among males in the 11 European countries where information on trends is available. Reported trends for women are less favourable, with 5 out of the 11 countries showing an increasing prevalence of smoking, albeit from initially low levels. Debates continue about the importance of dietary factors, such as greater consumption of animal fat in the development of cancer and a greater consumption of fibre in cancer prevention. Overexposure to sunlight is a growing problem *(61)*.

Considerable progress could be made in cancer control *(62)*. Ten Member States have a cancer policy or national plan, but not all of them are comprehensive and the priorities set in policy are not always reflected in programme activities and resource allocation. Only one quarter of the countries in the Region are fully covered by population-based cancer registries that provide the necessary foundation for planning, managing and evaluating cancer services. The resources available for cancer control are often inappropriately distributed because modern managerial techniques are not used in priority setting. Preventive health education has rarely been supplemented with legislative and regulatory measures that would make it more effective. The potential of screening for early detection has not been fully realized because of problems in organizing the service and lack of acceptance by the women for whom the service is intended. Excessive emphasis has been placed on providing treatment, and resources are often wasted on therapy that is ineffective, while palliative care and pain control, which would improve the quality of life for cancer patients, have been neglected. Properly trained health professionals with knowledge of treatment and supportive care practices are also scarce.

Suggested solutions   Every country should consider the potential benefits of comprehensive cancer control policies that make an explicit political commitment to improving prevention and treatment *(63)*. Such policies should define the objectives of comprehensive cancer control and the relative priority of each objective, and indicate the resources and measures required to attain these objectives. In many instances, this policy will be part of an overall plan for the prevention and control of noncommunicable disease.

A striking example of the benefits of a long-term commitment to cancer prevention can be found in the experience of one Member State *(64)*. Over the period 1970 – 1987, this country reduced cancer mortality in people under 65 by 22% through a combination of anti-smoking campaigns and intensive screening of specific groups.

Primary prevention   Strategies for implementation need to strike the appropriate balance between prevention, treatment and care. They can be based on information obtained from population-wide cancer registries, either covering the entire country or some suitable sample of different areas or regions. In most countries, the prevention of smoking should receive more attention than it does at present. Reduction of smoking, by preventing the recruitment of new smokers and helping existing smokers to stop, would be the most important contribution to the primary prevention of cancer (measures for smoking prevention are discussed under target 17) *(65)*. It would also reduce the incidence of other conditions, notably cardiovascular disease (target 9). Environmental initiatives such as reducing occupational exposure to asbestos (targets 21 and 25), preventing air pollution (target 21) and lowering iatrogenic exposure to X-rays will make an important contribution to a reduction in cancer incidence. Modifications in diet and changes in sexual and reproductive behaviour may also have a beneficial effect.

Screening   Evidence shows that mortality from cancer of the cervix and breast could be substantially reduced by regular screening followed by immediate treatment *(66,67)*. The greatest declines in cervical cancer mortality have occurred in countries that have complete registration of the eligible population combined with individual invitation for screening and follow-up programmes. Screening programmes must be accessible and acceptable to women and should include counselling services to deal sensitively with the consequences of false positive and false negative findings. Both scientific and cost considerations will be necessary to decide the periodicity of screening. Physicians and nurses engaged in primary care can play an important role in encouraging women to use such programmes. Intensive efforts should also be made to develop techniques for the early detection and treatment of other types of cancer. Screening methods for colorectal cancer are at present under investigation.

Care   The use of guidelines on the management of care *(68)* can help to ensure that people receive quality care throughout the health service system (see target 31). Higher priority also needs to be given to the organization and delivery of palliative care in the community, with attention to the timely movement of patients from intensive treatment to supportive care *(69)*. Voluntary organizations and self-help groups can play a major role in the rehabilitation of cancer patients. Pain control deserves more attention, with better training of health professionals and a review of drug legislation to make relevant pharmaceuticals more easily available in the community *(70)*. The quality of life of people with cancer must also be maintained. Monitoring is vital in all settings where people with cancer are undergoing treatment or palliative care.

Education, training and research More intensive efforts need to be made to spread current knowledge about diagnosis and treatment among health care personnel. Finally, emphasis should also be given to population-based research on cancer prevalence and to evaluating the effectiveness of cancer control measures.

Target 11 – Accidents

By the year 2000, injury, disability and death arising from accidents should be reduced by at least 25%.

This target can be achieved through:

- *joint action by the health, education, transport, law, engineering and industrial sectors to reduce accidents related to traffic, home, work, sports and leisure, giving priority to reducing by 25% death and injury in children and young people;*

- *rapid response to the health needs that arise during emergencies and disasters and their aftermath.*

Problem statement Accidents are a significant public health problem in the European Region, causing death, injury and prolonged disability. While the overall scale of mortality from accidents is known, fewer data are available on the extent of injury and prolonged disability. Accidents take a wide variety of forms including road accidents, drowning, fires and falls in the home, and poisoning by chemicals and medicine; they also occur in association with sports and leisure activities. They occur disproportionately among children, young people and the elderly. Unintentional injuries, in addition to causing severe human suffering, have enormous repercussions in lost productivity and medical care costs.

Road accidents Although the incidence of road injuries has declined by 18% since 1970, road accidents are still one of the main causes of death among young people, especially males. In 1985, around one third of all deaths in the age group 15 – 24 years were caused by road accidents. Alcohol use is known to be a significant factor in a large proportion of road accidents *(71)*.

Occupational accidents Occupational accidents are indicators of system failures at the workplace, with an estimated risk of 3 accidents per 100 working population per year, resulting in a mortality rate of 5.96 per 100 000 working population *(72)*.

Accidents and falls associated with the handling of equipment remain the largest cause of morbidity, accounting for millions of days of time lost from work and high health care costs. In many countries, accidents at work are decreasing because of improved safety measures. Nevertheless, the information needed to identify the factors that lead to occupational accidents, including exposure to unsafe products, is not always available.

Home and leisure accidents   Home and leisure accidents are known to be major causes of morbidity, particularly among children and the elderly *(73)*. The risk of poisoning varies from country to country, involving several different agents including medicines, household products and pesticides. Burns are also a common problem. The growing interest in physical fitness has increased the number of people participating in sports activities, with a consequent increase in the number of accidents.

Disasters   Emergency situations resulting from natural and man-made disasters are a significant problem, as they are unpredictable and affect many services. They always require the rapid provision of emergency health services. Chemical and radiation accidents also require rapid identification of the toxic agent involved and the application of appropriate countermeasures. The long-term effects of disasters are also significant. In addition to medical care and access to water and sanitation facilities, food and shelter may have to be restored while services may have to be provided to deal with the psychosocial problems associated with the disaster *(74 – 76)*.

Suggested solutions   Preventing accidents and reducing injuries require the combined efforts of many fields. Health, education, transport, urban planning and many branches of industry need to take intersectoral action based on strong advocacy led by the health sector (see target 37). In designing or modifying living and working environments, particular attention needs to be paid to eliminating and reducing hazards (see Chapter 5). Priority should be given to research into, and the achievement of, product safety through legislative controls, the use of standards and the appropriate use of economic incentives. Research is also needed on human behaviour patterns and accident psychology.

The consequences for individuals' health of accidents or disasters necessitate action to provide appropriate acute medical intervention, rehabilitation services, and support for those suffering long-term disability (see targets 3 and 4).

Road accidents   Many initiatives have been launched to improve the safety of transport. These include improving road networks, imposing speed limits, harmonizing the dimensions of vehicles, adding new safety features to vehicles, introducing seat belt regulations, and using education and the law to improve drivers' behaviour. Strong measures to prohibit drinking and driving are particularly important (see target 17). These initiatives have considerably reduced accidents and injuries. Traffic saturation on routes continues to be a problem, but can be eased by improvements in public transport networks. Population growth and industrial development in many European cities is causing congestion through competition for scarce space. Solutions to these problems will require progressive changes in the pattern of life in urban areas and, in some cases, regional planning will be needed to reverse the flow of population towards urban centres.

Occupational accidents While the number of accidents and injuries in the workplace is declining, the continued development of new technological processes will require a corresponding development of protection for the workforce. The role of occupational health services in tackling this problem is covered in target 25 *(77)*.

Home and leisure accidents In most cases, home accidents can be prevented by simple measures, but the general population needs to be more aware of how to make their homes safer places. Education and information campaigns will assist in this, and should be aimed particularly at the needs of children and the elderly. Rules to promote safe participation in sports and leisure activities need to be reinforced and implemented. Greater safety in sports can be achieved through the use of safer sports equipment, protective devices and better facilities.

Educational programmes on accident prevention must start early, for example with expectant parents and preschool children. This is crucial in view of the high number of accidents affecting children and because life-long values and behaviour patterns are formed, to a large extent, in early life.

Disasters To respond effectively to natural and man-made disasters, programmes need to be developed at the national, federal, regional and district levels to maintain a state of preparedness for disasters and to alleviate their consequences. These programmes must be intersectoral and should involve services such as health, environment, communications, transport and public information, to ensure coordinated management. They need to provide for a rapid response during both the emergency and the rehabilitation phases associated with disasters. Community health workers must be trained in areas where disasters are likely to occur, as well as in adjacent communities that may be affected by the disruption of the health infrastructure in the disaster area. The network of WHO collaborating centres for disaster preparedness needs to be reinforced. The centres' participation in training in preventive and mitigatory measures in Member States needs to be developed.

Target 12 – Reducing mental disorders and suicide

By the year 2000, there should be a sustained and continuing reduction in the prevalence of mental disorders, an improvement in the quality of life of all people with such disorders, and a reversal of the rising trends in suicide and attempted suicide.

This target can be achieved through:

- *improvement in societal factors, such as unemployment and social isolation, that put a strain on the individual;*

- *improved access to measures that support people and equip them to cope with distressing or stressful events and conditions;*

- *improved access to measures that support carers, both formal and informal, and people with mental disorders, especially dementia;*

- *development of comprehensive community-based mental health services with a greater involvement of primary health care;*

- *special efforts to prevent health-damaging types of behaviour such as substance abuse;*

- *programmes for suicide prevention.*

Problem statement   At least 5% of the population in the Region is estimated to suffer from serious diagnosable mental disorders (neuroses and functional psychoses), although prevalence estimates vary widely from study to study *(78 – 80)*. At least an additional 15% of the population is estimated to suffer less severe, but potentially incapacitating, forms of mental distress. These conditions affect social wellbeing and create the risk of more serious mental health problems and life-threatening behaviour such as suicide, violence and substance abuse.

Demographic trends in the European Region mean that dementia will become an increasing problem in the future, as the prevalence of dementia is strongly age-related. A meta-analysis of 47 studies *(81)* yielded average estimates of the prevalence of moderate or severe dementia of 1.4% for the 65 – 69 age group, rising to 38.6% for the 90 – 95 age group. Recent studies show the lowest estimates for these age groups to be 0.6% and 19% respectively *(82)*.

Conditions that increase people's vulnerability to mental distress are increasing. They include stressful lifestyles, prolonged unemployment, high mobility and weakening of family and social networks with resulting loss of social support and growing social isolation *(31)*. Current socioeconomic changes, particularly in the central and eastern part of the Region, add an additional dimension to these problems. Political change throughout the Region is likely to encourage greater migration in the future. Indicators of social violence, such as deaths from homicide and purposeful injury, are rising.

In most countries, suicide rates in 1988/1989 were higher than in 1970. Some countries that showed a significant increase in suicide rates during the 1970s and early 1980s are now experiencing a levelling off or a slight decline. In other countries, however, data for the late 1980s still show increasing trends. In 1985, suicide was the first, second or third most prevalent cause of death in adolescents and young adults, depending on the country. In the European Region as a whole, it accounted for 15% of deaths among males aged 15 – 24 and 19% among those aged 25 – 34, with rates of 12% and 14%, respectively, for females in the same age groups. In most countries, rates of suicide for those over 65 years of age are high compared with rates for other age groups. This will become an increasingly important problem as the population ages. Data on the incidence of attempted suicide and deliberate self-harm are not available on a complete or consistent basis throughout the Region. Reports from a number of centres suggest, however, that parasuicide, which is most prevalent among those aged 15 – 39, seems to have increased dramatically over the past two decades *(83,84)*, even taking into account the difficulties of interpreting data on parasuicide in different countries, cultures and religions.

Progress in moving from institutional care to flexible comprehensive community-based mental health services appears to be slow. Existing mental health services have not been well integrated with primary care provided through general practitioners or health centres, even where there is a stated intention to do so *(85)*. Increases in the number of mental health professionals with specialized training have not been accompanied by any development in coordinated approaches to care and integrated clinical practice, especially for those requiring long-term care. The reduction in the number of large mental hospitals is a positive trend in the Region, but the size of remaining mental hospitals continues to be large and they continue to operate alongside, rather than within, the general health care system. The number of psychiatric beds in general hospitals has grown by 50%, but it remains less than 10% of the total beds set aside for psychiatric care *(86)*.

Suggested solutions   Improvements in mental health will require the development of structures and mechanisms to support a comprehensive set of community-based services. Such services need to be made more accessible and appropriate and must actively reach out into the community. They should be based on policy, legislation and funding mechanisms that support their development. Mental health programmes need to be better coordinated with primary health care, public health and social services at the community level, and the staff involved need broader training (see target 28 on primary health care and target 30 on community services to meet special needs). The quality of life of people with mental disorders will have to be measured to assess the provision and quality of such services.

Quality of services   The development of more sensitive care for mentally ill people needs to be given priority. This will require a more holistic approach to the training of health and social care personnel, as well as better information for the public about available services. Efforts are required to continue the move from institutional to community-based care wherever possible (see target 29). The human rights and quality of life of people who are in hospital because of mental health problems must be maintained and protected. Several Member States have suitable monitoring systems: external observers or committees, set up with appropriate representation, have rights of visit and access to protect human rights in hospitals (see target 38). Representatives of people with mental disorders, their carers and voluntary organizations working in the field need to be actively involved in shaping the planning and provision of services.

Prevention   New and more widely available approaches are needed to equip people to deal with the distressing conditions associated with cultural and social change in society *(31)*. The discussion under the individual targets in Chapter 4 provides specific examples of measures that can be adopted. These include educational programmes to strengthen people's coping skills and preventive intervention for people facing crisis, unemployment or social isolation. They also include programmes that will strengthen both formal and informal social networks, as well as specific measures to provide support to people with mental health problems, and to their carers, both formal and informal. The services involved must be made available in primary care settings. An important primary prevention measure is to design living and working environments with mental and social needs in mind and provide settings that help to break down social isolation and encourage participation in community life (see targets 24 and 25). Because of their growing numbers, the particular needs of migrants, the unemployed and other vulnerable groups in the population require priority attention.

Suicide   Reversing trends in suicide rates will require national or federal and local programmes for suicide prevention. At least one Member State has already started implementing a comprehensive national programme, the first stages of which involved research and the planning of strategy. Practical preventive programmes have now begun and will be followed up and evaluated. Better coordination is particularly important between mental health services and those provided by general hospitals, primary care services, substance abuse services and voluntary groups. Information on effective approaches needs to be more widely disseminated, and monitoring and research need to be improved. The role of the media also needs attention *(83)*.

Substance abuse   Special efforts are needed to prevent the problems associated with health-damaging behaviour such as substance abuse. At present, a health promotion approach, directed at educating families and strengthening the skills of young people, appears to be the most realistic means of affecting positively the formation of relevant attitudes and behaviours at an early stage in life. The role of families, schools and preschool education in this process will be decisive. Services for mental health and for drug and alcohol abuse also need to be more closely integrated at the local level. Specific examples of approaches that can be used are discussed further under target 17 (tobacco, alcohol and psychoactive drugs) and other targets in Chapter 4.

Research   International comparative research into the causes, consequences and incidence of mental disease and mental distress will help improve the planning and provision of services for the future.

References

1. *Monitoring of the strategy for health for all by the year 2000. Part 1: the situation in the European Region, 1987/1988.* Copenhagen, WHO Regional Office for Europe, 1989 (document EUR/HST/89.1).
2. *Implementation of the global strategy for health for all by the year 2000, second evaluation: eighth report on the world health situation. Volume 5. European Region.* Copenhagen, WHO Regional Office for Europe, 1993 (WHO Regional Publications, European Series, No. 52).
3. TOWNSEND, P. & DAVIDSON, N., ED. The Black report. *In: Inequalities in health.* Harmondsworth, Penguin, 1992.

4. *La santé en France. Rapport au Ministre des affaires sociales et de la solidarité nationale et au Secrétaire d'Etat chargé de la santé.* Paris, La documentation française, 1985.

5. LECLERC, A. ET AL. Differential mortality. Some comparisons between England and Wales, Finland and France based on inequality measures. *International journal of epidemiology*, **19**(4): 1001 – 1010 (1990).

6. JOZAN, P. *An ecological approach in revealing socioeconomic differentials in mortality: some preliminary results of the Budapest Mortality Study*. Budapest, Hungarian Central Statistical Office, 1984.

7. MARMOT, M. Socioeconomic determinants of CHD mortality. *International journal of epidemiology*, **18**(Suppl. 1): S196 – S202 (1989).

8. *Movimiento nacional de la población 1979* [National population trends 1979]. Madrid, Instituto Nacional de Estadistica, 1981.

9. WHITEHEAD, M. The health divide. *In*: *Inequalities in health*. Harmondsworth, Penguin, 1992.

10. ILLSLEY, R. & SVENSSON, P., ED. Health inequities in Europe. *Social science and medicine*, **31**(3): 233 – 420 (1990).

11. WNUK-LIPINSKI, E. & ILLSLEY, R. Non-market economies in health. Introduction. *Social science and medicine*, **31**(8): 833 – 836 (1990).

12. FOX, J., ED. *Health inequalities in European countries*. London, Gower, 1989.

13. GUNNING-SCHEPERS, L. ET AL., ED. *Socioeconomic inequalities in health: questions on trends and explanations*. The Hague, Ministry of Welfare, Health and Cultural Affairs, 1989.

14. KALIMO, E. ET AL. *Need, use and expenses of health services in Finland, 1964 – 1976*. Helsinki, Social Insurance Institution, 1983.

15. WHITEHEAD, M. *The concepts and principles of equity and health*. Copenhagen, WHO Regional Office for Europe, 1990 (document EUR/ICP/RPD 414).

16. DAHLGREN, G. & WHITEHEAD, M. *Policies and strategies to promote equity in health*. Copenhagen, WHO Regional Office for Europe, 1992 (document EUR/ICP/RPD 414(2)).

17. STARRIN, B. ET AL., ED. *Unemployment, poverty and quality of working life: some European experiences*. Berlin, Edition Sigma, 1989.

18. GUPTA, S. *The mental health problems of migrants: report from six European countries*. Copenhagen, WHO Regional Office for Europe, 1991 (document EUR/ICP/PSF 034(A)).

19. *Improving the quality of life by reducing chronic (nonmalignant) pain*: report on a WHO Consultation. Copenhagen, WHO Regional Office for Europe, 1992 (document EUR/ICP/RHB 024).

20. KAPLUN, A., ED. *Health promotion and chronic illness; discovering a new quality of health*. Copenhagen, WHO Regional Office for Europe, 1992 (WHO Regional Publications, European Series, No. 44).

21. *Approaches to stress management in the community setting*: report on a WHO Consultation. Copenhagen, WHO Regional Office for Europe, 1992 (document EUR/ICP/PSF 028).

22. ABIVEN, M. Dying with dignity. *World health forum*, **12**: 375 – 399 (1991).

23. FALLOWFIELD, L. *The quality of life: the missing measurement in health care*. London, Souvenir Press, 1990.

24. BOWLING, A. *Measuring health, a review of quality of life measurement scales*. Buckingham, Open University Press, 1992.

25. HAYS, R.D. & SHAPIRO, M.F. An overview of generic health-related quality of life measures for HIV research. *Quality of life research*, **1**: 91 – 97 (1992).

26. KAPLAN, R.K. & ANDERSON, J.P. The general health policy model: an integrated approach. *In*: Spiker. B., ed. *Quality of life assessments in clinical trials*. New York, Raven Press, 1990.

27. KIND, P. *The design and construction of quality of life measures*. York, University of York, Health Economics Consortium, Centre for Health Economics, 1988 (Discussion Paper No. 43).

28. Quality of life and life satisfaction (Chapter 6) and General health measurements (Chapter 8). *In*: McDowell, I. & Newell, C., ed. *Measuring health: a guide to rating scales and questionnaires*. Oxford, Oxford University Press, 1987.

29. BRADLEY, C., ED. *Handbook of psychology and diabetes*: a guide to psychological measurement in diabetes research and practice. Reading, Harwood Academic Publishers (in press).

30. WATERS, W.E. ET AL., ED. *Health, lifestyles and services for the elderly*. Copenhagen, WHO Regional Office for Europe, 1989 (Public Health in Europe, No. 29).

31. *Prevention of mental, psychosocial and neurological disorders in the European Region*. Copenhagen, WHO Regional Office for Europe, 1988 (document EUR/PSF/88.1).

32. LEPARSKI, E. & NÜSSEL, E., ED. *Protocol and guidelines for monitoring and evaluation procedures*. Berlin, Springer Verlag, 1987.

33. *Positioning CINDI to meet the challenges. The WHO CINDI policy framework for non-communicable disease prevention*: report of the Working Group on Policy Development. Copenhagen, WHO Regional Office for Europe, 1992 (document EUR/ICP/NCD 216).

34. *It can be done. A smoke-free Europe*. Copenhagen, WHO Regional Office for Europe, 1988 (WHO Regional Publications, European Series, No. 30).

35. Diabetes Care and Research in Europe: the St Vincent declaration. *Diabetic medicine*, 7: 360 (1990).

36. MODELL, B. ET AL. *Community genetics services in Europe*. Copenhagen, WHO Regional Office for Europe, 1991 (WHO Regional Publications, European Series, No. 38).

37. *Expanded Programme on Immunization and related activities in Europe*: progress report. Copenhagen, WHO Regional Office for Europe, 1985 (document EUR/RC35/8).

38. *Expanded Programme on Immunization*: progress report. Copenhagen, WHO Regional Office for Europe, 1990 (document EUR/RC40/12).

39. *Seventh meeting of the European Advisory Group (EAG) on the Expanded programme on Immunization (EPI)*. Copenhagen, WHO Regional Office for Europe, 1993 (document EUR/ICP/EPI 012/B).

40. *AIDS surveillance in Europe*. Paris, European Centre for Epidemiological Monitoring of AIDS, 1991 (Quarterly Report No. 32).

41. *Pneumonia in children in Europe*: report on a WHO meeting. Copenhagen, WHO Regional Office for Europe, 1991 (document EUR/ICP/ARI 012).

42. *Psychosocial aspects of HIV and AIDS and the evaluation of preventive strategies*: report on a WHO meeting. Copenhagen, WHO Regional Office for Europe, 1990 (WHO Regional Publications, European Series, No. 36).

43. ROTT, C. & OSWALD, F., ED. *Kompetenz im Alter. Beiträge zur III. Gerontologischen Woche, Heidelberg, 2. – 6. Mai 1988*. Vaduz, Liechtenstein Verlag AG, 1989.

44. HEIKKINEN, E. ET AL. *The elderly in eleven countries: a sociomedical survey*. Copenhagen, WHO Regional Office for Europe, 1983 (Public Health in Europe, No. 21).

45. *Convention on the Rights of the Child*. Geneva, UNICEF/United Nations Centre for Human Rights, 1989.

46. *SIDS: a report on current knowledge and research recommendations*. Washington, DC, Department of Health and Human Services, 1989.

47. *Young Europeans, tobacco and alcohol: a survey in the 12 member states of the EC among young people aged 11 to 15*. Brussels, Commission of the European Communities, 1990.

48. *The health of Canada's youth. Views and behaviours of 11-, 13- and 15-year-olds from 11 countries*. Ottawa, Health and Welfare Canada, 1992.

49. *International Code of Marketing of Breast-milk Substitutes*. Geneva, World Health Organization, 1981.

50. *Lactation management training*. Copenhagen, WHO Regional Office for Europe, 1991 (document EUR/ICP/NUT 138).

51. DRAIJER, J. & WILLIAMS, T. *School health education and promotion in the member states of the European Community*. Luxembourg, Commission of the European Communities, 1991.

52. YOUNG, I. & WILLIAMS, T. *The healthy school*. Edinburgh, Scottish Health Education Group, 1989.

53. *European network of health-promoting schools – resource pack*. Copenhagen, WHO Regional Office for Europe, 1992 (document).

54. SHAFER, M.A. & SWEET, R.L. Pelvic inflammatory disease in adolescent females. *Pediatric clinics of North America*, **36**(3): 513 – 532 (1989).

55. BURNAKIS, T.G. & HILDEBRANDT, N.B. Pelvic inflammatory disease: a review with emphasis on antimicrobial therapy. *Reviews of infectious diseases*, **8**(1): 86 – 116 (1986).

56. BLAXTER, M. Evidence on inequality in health from a national survey. *Lancet*, **2**: 30 – 33 (1987).

57. The Adelaide recommendations: healthy public policy. *Health promotion*, **3**(2): 183 – 186 (1988).

58. *National agenda for women. Mid-term implementation report on the 1988 – 92 five-year action plans*. Canberra, Australian Government Publishing Service, 1990.

59. *National Policy on Women's Health: a framework for change*. Canberra, Australian Government Publishing Service, 1988.

60. *Positive approaches to promoting women's health*. Copenhagen, WHO Regional Office for Europe, 1985 (document ICP/HSR/603/s01).

61. VAN OYEN, H. & DÖBRÖSSY, L. Cancer experience in the European Region, 1970 through 1985. *European journal of public health* (in press).

62. DÖBRÖSSY, L. *Statement on the status of cancer and cancer control in Europe*. Copenhagen, WHO Regional Office for Europe, 1990 (document EUR/ICP/CAN 115(2)).

63. *Cancer control programming in the European Region of the World Health Organization. Guideline document*. Copenhagen, WHO Regional Office for Europe, 1985 (document ICP/CAN 101).

64. *Cancer in Finland in 1954 – 2008. Incidence, mortality and prevalence*. Helsinki, Finnish Cancer Registry, 1989.

65. *Cancer: causes, occurrence and control*. Lyon, International Agency for Research on Cancer, 1991 (IARC Scientific Publications, No. 100).

66. LAARA, E. ET AL. Trends in mortality from cervical cancer in the Nordic countries: association with organized screening programmes. *Lancet*, **1**: 1247 – 1249 (1987).

67. TABOR, L. ET AL. Reduction in mortality from breast cancer after mass screening with mammography. *Lancet*, **1**: 829 – 832 (1988).

68. *Development of care programmes for cancer.* Guideline document. Copenhagen, WHO Regional Office for Europe, 1986 (document ICP/CAN 119).

69. *Palliative cancer care*: policy statement based on the recommendations of a WHO consultation. Copenhagen, WHO Regional Office for Europe, 1989.

70. WHO Technical Report Series, No. 804, 1990 (*Cancer pain relief and palliative care*: report of a WHO Expert Committee).

71. *Alcohol and accidents.* London, British Medical Association, 1989.

72. RANTANEN, J., ED. *Occupational health services: an overview.* Copenhagen, WHO Regional Office for Europe, 1990 (WHO Regional Publications, European Series, No. 26).

73. BISTRUP, M.L. *Housing and community environments. How they support health.* Copenhagen, National Board of Health, 1991 (Briefing book for the Sundsvall Conference on Supportive Environments).

74. *Psychological effects of nuclear accidents*: report on a WHO Working Group. Copenhagen, WHO Regional Office for Europe, 1990 (document EUR/ICP/CEH 093(S)).

75. *Psychosocial consequences of disasters: prevention and management.* Geneva, World Health Organization, 1992 (document WHO/MNH/PSF91.3).

76. *Red Cross/Red Crescent response to meeting the psychological needs resulting from stressful life events and disasters*: report on a consultation. Copenhagen, Danish Red Cross, 1991.

77. *Work for health?* Stockholm, National Board of Health and Welfare, 1991 (Briefing book for the Sundsvall Conference on Supportive Environments).

78. FURER, J.W. & TAX, B., ED. *Somatische klachten, psychiatrische symptomen en psychosociale problemen. Eindrapport van het Regioproject Nijmegen, deel I* [Somatic complaints, psychiatric symptoms and psychosocial problems. Final report on the Nijmegen Regional Project, part I]. Nijmegen, Institute of Social Medicine, Nijmegen Catholic University, 1987.

79. HODIAMONT, P.P.G. *Het zoeken van zieke zielen* [Seeking sick souls]. Thesis, Nijmegen Catholic University, 1986.

80. STEERING COMMITTEE ON FUTURE HEALTH SCENARIOS. *Caring for mental health in the future.* Dordrecht, Kluwer Academic Publishers, 1992.

81. JORM, A.F. ET AL. The prevalence of dementia: a quantitative integration of the literature. *Acta psychiatrica scandinavica*, **76**: 465 – 479 (1987).

82. O'CONNOR, D.W. ET AL. The prevalence of dementia as measured by the Cambridge Mental Disorders of Elderly Dementia. *Acta psychiatrica scandinavica*, **79**: 190 – 198 (1989).

83. *Strategies for reducing suicidal behaviour in the European Region*: report on a WHO consultation. Copenhagen, WHO Regional Office for Europe, 1990 (document EUR/ICP/PSF 024(S)).

84. Parasuicide in Europe: the WHO/EURO multicentre study on parasuicide, I. Introduction and preliminary analysis for 1989. *Acta psychiatrica scandinavica*, **85**(2): 97 – 104 (1992).

85. *Mental health services in pilot study areas*: report on a European study. Copenhagen, WHO Regional Office for Europe, 1987.

86. FREEMAN, H.L. ET AL. *Mental health services in Europe: 10 years on.* Copenhagen, WHO Regional Office for Europe, 1985 (Public Health in Europe, No. 25).

4

Lifestyles conducive to health

Lifestyles depend on the values, priorities, practical opportunities and constraints that people experience in daily life. The lifestyles of societies, social groups and individuals overlap to create recurring patterns of action. Attitudes, competence and behaviours that influence health are shaped by this experience and the social meanings inferred from it. They are not merely rational decisions to accept or avoid health risks. This means that healthy lifestyles have to be promoted as realistic and attractive alternatives that people can, in fact, act upon. "To make the healthy choice the easier choice", one of the guiding principles of the health for all philosophy and especially of health promotion, means creating opportunities for people to take practical action.

Since 1984, when the European health for all targets were adopted, public interest in positive health, in healthy ways of living and eating, and in physical and mental wellbeing has increased in the European Region. This trend has been supported by media interest in health issues and in the spread of health promotion programmes. Although many factors may have influenced this development, the strong lifestyle and health component of the European health for all policy and the corresponding Regional Office programme must surely have played an important part in raising awareness and motivation.

In most countries, however, successes in lifestyle change have been confined largely to the middle strata of society, where socially and economically privileged people have greater opportunities to live healthy lives. Disadvantaged people who face basic problems in their daily lives have less time and fewer resources to devote to healthy lifestyles and environmental concerns. Practices that are harmful to health, such as smoking and excessive use of alcohol, tend to occur more frequently among people with low incomes, partly as a means of coping with stress. The resulting inequitable access to health remains a major challenge for health policy. It puts some individuals and families at a disadvantage, and results in high costs to society.

The Ottawa Charter: a strategy for health promotion The relationships between lifestyles, environment and health are complex, as are the impacts of policies that shape them. In conceptual terms, they are expressed as multidimensional models that can be difficult to translate directly into action. The Ottawa Charter for Health Promotion *(1)*, adopted at a WHO conference in 1986, addresses this challenge. It stresses a new health for all mandate for the health sector that goes beyond traditional health services. It emphasizes health rather than illness. This new health mandate has three key features. It aims to enable people to reach their full health potential; it encourages advocacy for health; and it seeks to mediate conflicting interests in society so as to support health development.

The Charter has set a new direction for health promotion by defining a comprehensive, but straightforward, strategy with five components: healthy public policy, supportive environments, personal skills, community action and reoriented health services.

Building healthy public policy   Policies that shape the economic and social conditions under which people live also create opportunities and incentives for them to select or reject healthy patterns of living. The policies of governments and of the private corporations that control the production and promotion of certain consumer goods affect lifestyles in ways that are at times harmful. Target 1 (equity in health) addresses the link between poverty and ill health. The promotion of health through lifestyle changes can only be effective if the political and societal resolve exists to improve the overall standard of living.

Healthy public policy *(2)* provides the foundation for promoting physical and social environments that support the adoption of healthy patterns of living. Its aim is to ensure equitable access to the prerequisites for health, whether in the form of consumer goods, supportive living environments or services that contribute to healthy living. It helps to make healthy choices the easy choices. Decision-makers at all levels and in all sectors must be aware of the consequences for health of their decisions. They must also be willing to accept their share of responsibility for health in their communities.

Ethical issues must be considered when healthy public policies are being devised. A delicate balance must be achieved between respect for the individual's right to free choice and the duty of society to promote the health of its population.

Creating supportive environments   Health is created in the context of everyday life. The environments of work, learning, leisure and family life must be health enhancing. Supportive environments have both physical and social dimensions. A strategy for creating supportive environments must strengthen the social support systems that are offered by families, friends, self-help groups and other social networks. These can provide benefits in everyday life as well as support in adverse circumstances, such as unemployment and migration *(3,4)*.

In many areas, urbanization and technological development are rapidly changing the environment. Such changes can present opportunities to influence events in the interest of the promotion of health. Fortunately, public concern for the protection of natural, built and social environments is becoming stronger, as is concern for the conservation of resources. This provides an essential bridge between environmental conservation and the promotion of health.

Developing personal skills Strengthening people's capacity to make personal choices and cope with stressful situations is a formidable challenge for modern society. Self-esteem is an essential part of a person's ability to apply health knowledge and choose a healthy lifestyle. Health education must particularly emphasize personal and social development and the building of health competence. Recognition of the importance of personal skills as a basis for a healthy lifestyle is leading to a new emphasis in health education on empowerment. This means developing people's skills and highlighting their options so that they can exercise more control over their lives.

Strengthening community action Communities in modern society do not always define themselves through physical proximity. Many arise around common issues or causes, such as self-help groups and environmental conservation.

Involving communities in setting priorities, making decisions and taking action lies at the heart of effective health promotion. Successful initiatives throughout the European Region have been based on this principle, for example in cardiovascular disease and in women's health.

Community-based health promotion strategies have several benefits. They draw on existing human and material resources while strengthening people's sense of self-worth, widening their knowledge base and expertise, and providing them with an avenue for social support. They create a sustainable and adaptable resource, sensitive to social and cultural values.

Reorienting health services Health for all urges the whole of the health service sector to move towards health promotion. This means that health care must include a focus on health and disease prevention. Organizational changes are now taking place in several countries in the Region to embrace an expanded mandate in health promotion, to emphasize disease prevention in primary care, to include health education as part of patient services in hospitals, and to strengthen health care facilities as settings that promote health.

Health services are major employers. Their staff form an important reference group for the rest of the community. Their active participation in health promotion and their own example can therefore be of added benefit to the whole population.

Sickness insurance funds, where they exist, can also be involved in health promotion and disease prevention programmes.

Five interrelated targets The targets in this chapter weave together the five components of the Ottawa Charter to create a comprehensive approach to the support of positive changes in living patterns. This can be characterized as an environmental approach in that it explicitly recognizes the constraints and impacts of physical, economic, social and cultural environments on the choices and actions of individuals and groups. It seeks to promote health by modifying such constraints and influences as well as by working with individuals. The targets require the mobilization and motivation of a wide range of partners, both inside and outside the health sector, as advocates for health and as mediators between differing interests in society. They also require widespread efforts to empower individuals and groups to exercise more control over their lives and their health. The targets emphasize health promotion, intersectoral action and community participation, which are key principles of the health for all strategy.

Fig. 3 groups the targets of the chapter into policy, action and outcome. Target 13, on healthy public policy, calls on both the public and the private sectors to adopt policies that will support health. The implementation of such policies will provide the basis for the changes sought in target 14, which focuses on developing opportunities for health promotion in all the settings of daily life: workplaces, schools, homes, neighbourhoods and cities. Target 15 deals with the need to develop public and professional competence in health, including effective health education for the general population supported by well informed and trained health professionals, and the need to increase health awareness in other sectors. The last two targets address effective health promotion. Target 16 is concerned with healthy patterns of living. Target 17 deals with reductions in the health-damaging consumption of substances, such as alcohol, tobacco and drugs, that create dependence.

Fig. 3. Lifestyles conducive to health

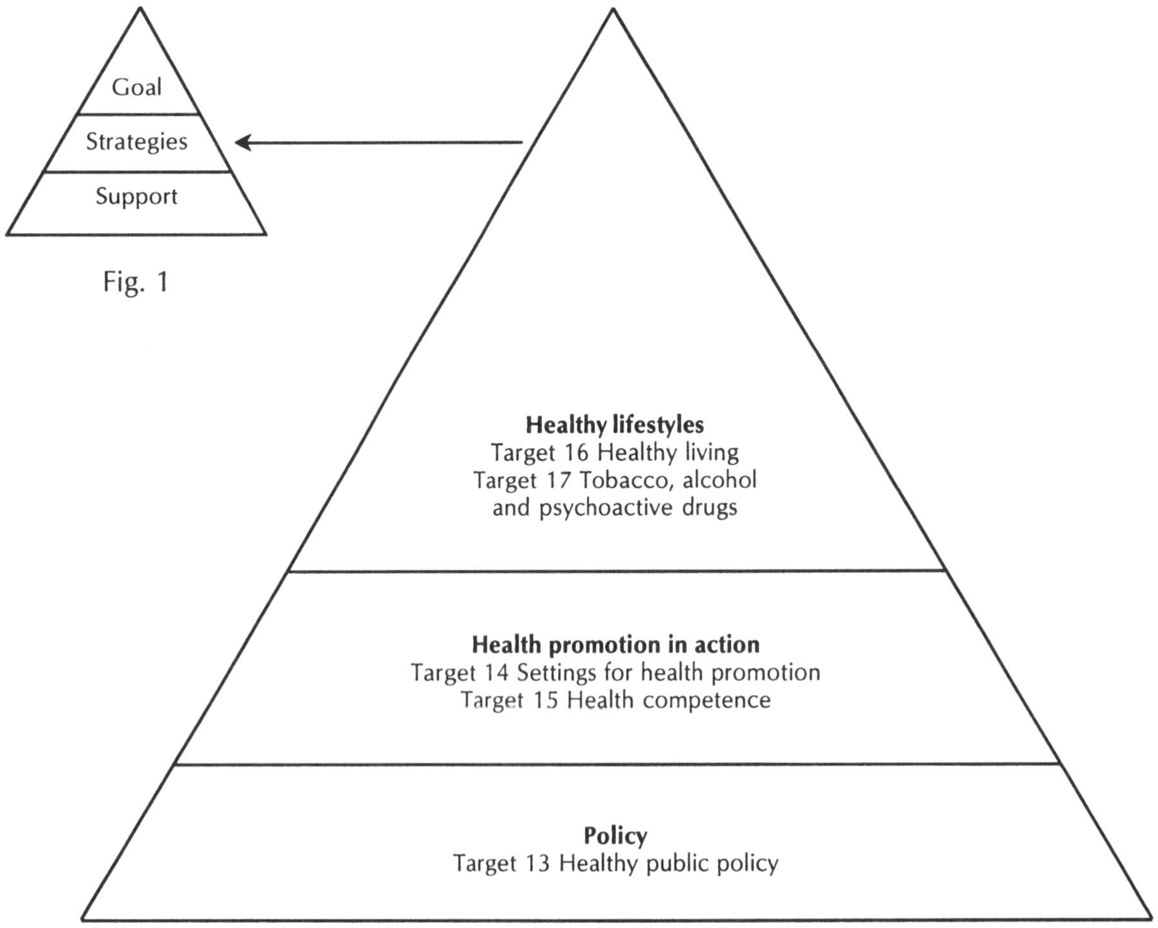

Goal
Strategies
Support

Fig. 1

Healthy lifestyles
Target 16 Healthy living
Target 17 Tobacco, alcohol
and psychoactive drugs

Health promotion in action
Target 14 Settings for health promotion
Target 15 Health competence

Policy
Target 13 Healthy public policy

Target 13 – Healthy public policy

By the year 2000, all Member States should have developed, and be implementing, intersectoral policies for the promotion of healthy lifestyles, with systems ensuring public participation in policy-making and implementation.

This target can be achieved if:

- *policies are formulated as an essential component of health for all policy in Member States and are continuously updated and developed;*

- *the impact on health of existing public policies in all sectors is periodically assessed;*

- *mechanisms are being used at country, regional and local levels to involve people in policy-making and implementation;*

- *effective mechanisms are being used at country, regional and local levels to support intersectoral action;*

- *legislative, financial and administrative support for health promotion is strengthened and investment in health increased;*

- *indicators are developed to provide the basis for monitoring progress towards healthy patterns of living.*

Problem statement Commitment to healthy public policy varies significantly between Member States. Where progress is being made, it is often fragmentary and half-hearted. The rapid pace of social, economic and political change, particularly in central and eastern parts of the Region, risks eroding any progress that has been made because of economic scarcity, fiscal upheaval and political transition. There is a gross imbalance in the influence on policy exercised on the one hand by several powerful and wealthy interest groups, such as the tobacco and food industries, and on the other by those concerned with public health. For some products, such as tobacco, WHO's attempts to develop an international consensus on policy have been supported by the European Community, but such cooperation needs further strengthening. Effective means to ensure consumer involvement in policy development do not exist in many Member States.

The economic and political priorities of countries are often inconsistent with progress towards healthy public policy. Recent WHO conferences have exposed this conflict, including the European Conference on Tobacco Policy *(5)* held in Madrid in

1988, and the European Conference on Food and Nutrition Policy (6) in Budapest in 1990. Several areas of policy conflict are now widely recognized.

First, government subsidies are used to support the production of unhealthy products. Under the Common Agricultural Policy, for example, the European Community has subsidized tobacco and alcohol production as well as a range of less than desirable food products. The current estimated value of these subsidies for tobacco alone is about US $1500 million (7).

Second, controls on the advertising of unhealthy products such as alcohol and tobacco are inadequate in most countries. In one country (8), the tobacco industry was recently estimated to be spending more than US $300 million per year to promote smoking. This amounted to about US $6 for each person in the country.

Third, products officially considered dangerous and unhealthy in one country are often exported to other countries, particularly developing ones. Examples of such products are tobacco with high tar content, dairy and animal produce with a high concentration of fat, and hazardous pharmaceuticals.

Fourth, the pricing and taxation of consumer products often work against healthy choices. While alcohol and tobacco have often been priced at high levels to discourage consumption, these prices do not always keep pace with inflation. At the same time, products and services that contribute to health, such as fresh fruit and vegetables, non-alcoholic drinks, exercise facilities and contraceptives, are not subsidized enough to promote easy access. This results in the purchase of less healthy products, especially among lower income families.

Fifth, urban planning and construction practices often fail to recognize the need to create environments that are safe, accessible and conducive to social interaction and physical activity. Insufficient green space is allowed for play and recreation, the needs of car drivers are placed before the convenience and wellbeing of pedestrians and cyclists, and urban renewal projects often ignore the importance of maintaining socially cohesive neighbourhoods.

Suggested solutions   The effective formulation and implementation of healthy public policy require the creativity, resources and commitment of many people, including the general public, those in government, business, industry and the media, and professional groups. Legislative, financial and administrative support are also needed if health promotion is to be strengthened (2,9).

Countries with market economies (or moving towards such structures) must see public policy for health as an investment, with a considerable long-term pay-off in both social and economic terms. Countries reforming their economic structure to decentralize commercial planning and organizational management need to make special efforts to ensure that the benefits and methods of healthy public policy are made widely known to decision-makers throughout the political and economic system.

The growing public concern about wellbeing, environment and ecology and the increasing activity of consumer groups provide the support needed to begin progress towards healthy public policy. The active involvement of the community is crucial; without it, healthy public policy will not receive the popular and political support it needs. Politicians and other decision-makers in all sectors need to be highly conscious of the impact their decisions have on people's health. Better information and health impact analysis will help support this process, as will investment in research and in the dissemination of up-to-date knowledge.

A comprehensive examination of the health needs, capacities and prerequisites of population groups is the most effective approach to the development of healthy public policy. The population targets in Chapter 3 address groups that must receive urgent attention if equity in health is to be achieved. The settings approach described in target 14 provides a decentralized strategy for implementing healthy public policy.

Knowledge is growing rapidly about the organizational structures and management systems that support the formulation and implementation of healthy public policy. Five years ago, this experience was limited to national or federal government organizations, but it has now become much more widely available at regional and local levels. National and federal experience has mainly been gained with policies that influence access to consumer products such as food, tobacco and alcohol. This experience illustrates the importance of establishing mechanisms that ensure continuity in policy development, maintain the interest of policy-makers and consolidate gains that are achieved. Experience also shows the importance of developing comprehensive strategies that reinforce each other and of providing adequate opportunity to consult all who have an interest in the policy outcome, including the general public, producers and manufacturers.

Experience with the processes of policy formulation at the local level has been gained through the

WHO Healthy Cities project and the networks within countries associated with it. Coordinating committees that direct the projects bring together city politicians, municipal department heads and major interest groups in the community. They generate information and awareness and search for opportunities for innovative projects, such as strengthening the health aspect of urban redevelopment. Information exchange, the building of networks, advice and financial support have been used as incentives for project development.

Europe is a long way from applying the concepts of healthy public policy comprehensively and consistently in all sectors. A growing number of examples can be used, however, to explain the concept, explore its practical implications and demonstrate the creative use of policy opportunities.

First, information to help consumers make healthy choices can be made more accessible and appropriate. Health education authorities have been producing such material for some time. In some places consumer groups and business are now taking on the responsibility of doing so. In some Member States, the role of sickness insurance funds includes informing the people they insure about hazards to health in general and how to avoid them, and about disease prevention. Food labels are being used to identify levels of fat, sugar, salt and additives in products. Restrictions on tobacco and alcohol advertising are widespread and, in some Member States, standard rotating health warnings are printed on cigarette packets.

Second, environmental controls can help to ensure public access to safe products and environments. Standards of water, air and food quality have been adopted throughout the Region (see Chapter 5). In several countries, car seat belts have become mandatory. Prohibition of smoking in public areas and workplaces is becoming more common.

Third, taxation and financial incentives can be used to protect the environment, improve access to public facilities and encourage healthy consumer patterns. Environmental protection is encouraged by subsidies for public transport and for the production of unleaded petrol. Access to buildings can be made easier for people with disabilities through subsidies for the renovation of housing and public buildings. Tobacco and alcohol are taxed at high levels in several Member States to discourage their use and, in some cases, these revenues are used to finance health promotion.

Fourth, public financing can be used creatively to improve access to services for health promotion and disease prevention. In several countries, self-help initiatives in health promotion are supported through financial and/or other resources from the public health service. In one country, revenues obtained from sickness insurance funds are being used to finance health promotion in the workplace *(10)*.

One of the major challenges of the next decade will be to apply the experience gained in the development and implementation of healthy public policy to a wider array of situations in more Member States and communities. For this to happen, policy analysis and evaluative research will be required to capture the knowledge that is available, coupled with coordinated dissemination and training efforts to spread this knowledge throughout Member States and in different sectors.

Target 14 – Settings for health promotion

By the year 2000, all settings of social life and activity, such as the city, school, workplace, neighbourhood and home, should provide greater opportunities for promoting health.

This can be achieved if in all Member States action is taken in line with certain concepts and principles, such as those of the WHO Healthy Cities network, including steps to strengthen opportunities for health promotion in the various settings by:

- *concentrating health promotion on settings of daily living;*

- *facilitating community participation in decisions regarding health and the environment and health promotion;*

- *fostering cooperation between sectors, to create better opportunities for healthy living;*

- *encouraging the involvement of various disciplines in health promotion.*

Problem statement   Much disease, disability and premature death would not occur if settings where people live and work gave greater support for healthy living. The settings approach to health promotion uses decentralized strategies that aim to make the physical and social settings where people spend their lives contribute to their health. Homes, schools, workplaces and recreation areas can all make major contributions that complement each other. They can minimize risks to health in the environment; facilitate social interaction and break down social isolation; and incorporate activities that contribute to the promotion of health.

Problems in the physical environment that undermine health have become widely recognized over the past decade. The challenge that exists throughout the Region is particularly important in the central and eastern part. Acute problems of air, noise and water pollution and inadequate waste disposal make healthy living impossible. The differences between wealthy suburbs and deteriorating inner city neighbourhoods are increasing. Many schools are unhealthy places for children. Employers often do little to protect the safety or promote the health of their employees.

The social environment with all of its complexity is also a major factor in health. Households in the Region range from multiple generations of relatives living together to individuals living alone. Widespread migration disrupts family units and other social support systems. Feelings of alienation and powerlessness are growing, especially among minority groups and people with low incomes. Social and health services are often inflexible and insensitive to changing social realities and special needs. This has a serious impact on those who are most vulnerable.

Major contributions to health promotion can be incorporated into everyday activities. Every effort must be made to take advantage of the opportunities presented in this way.

Suggested solutions   Promoting healthy settings for living is the strategy for implementing healthy public policy at the local level. Four principles must be respected when developing such strategies. The strategies should:

– enable individuals and communities to exercise greater freedom to act in the interest of their own health;
– mediate between the conflicting interests of various groups and organizations involved in creating better health;
– facilitate the political, social, community and organizational processes used to arrive at new structures and methods for planning and decision-making;
– create new partnerships and coalitions for health that bring together different professional groups and sectors, united in the common purpose of promoting health.

The challenge is to offer incentives and support for the creation of settings where physical characteristics and social processes interact to enhance healthy living. Housing and neighbourhoods can be designed to strengthen the supporting and caring functions of families and friends. Schools and recreation areas can encourage social experiences that shape and maintain healthy behaviour among children. Workplaces can be safe and offer opportunities to be productive in an environment that encourages healthy lifestyles. Health centres and hospitals can be designed and organized to encourage an interest in health and offer models of healthy living. The city environment can offer older people and those with disabilities opportunities to live independently and participate actively in community life. Activities to strengthen personal skills and competence and provide relevant knowledge can be incorporated into the social interactions that take place in all the settings of daily life. Vulnerable and disadvantaged groups have limited access to services and education provided outside the normal settings of their daily lives. Health promotion and health education need to operate on an outreach basis if such groups are to be successfully targeted.

Promoting settings for healthy living requires action that cuts across traditional departmental lines and demands the creativity and resources of organizations in both the public and the private sectors. The achievement of equity, sustainable development and social mobility cannot be adequately addressed by any single organization acting alone. The challenge is to foster a new organizational and managerial culture that will break down the barriers and establish trust between sectors to facilitate a more comprehensive approach to solving problems.

Many players – including city planners and social workers, housing and traffic administrators, teachers and environmental officers, business employers and community activists – will have to be involved in health promotion that has a settings perspective. Structures will have to be created that bring community groups, organizations and professional disciplines together. The complex, interrelated nature of physical and social influences on health will need to be more clearly understood, explained and addressed in decision-making. This will require new ways of providing information and training for different professional

groups. Flexible forms of project management that share resources and facilitate cooperative decision-making will have to be used.

The active involvement of people is a major factor in the success of a settings approach to health promotion. The people who live, learn and work in the settings where health is being promoted must be actively involved in deciding what those settings will be like. People in positions of responsibility must give fewer directives and spend more time and energy on negotiation. A variety of structures and processes will be needed to encourage and allow people to arrive at their own definition of issues that are important for their health, make plans to deal with them, and work actively towards their implementation.

Strategies for strengthening the contribution of physical settings to health are highly developed in the Region. The European Charter on Environment and Health (11), adopted in Frankfurt in 1989, provides a framework for such strategies. Measures to prevent the pollution of air, water and soil and to improve waste management, all critical health issues, are addressed by targets in Chapter 5, as are measures to make urban and rural settlements more supportive of health, and to promote the health and wellbeing of people at work.

Programmes that will facilitate social interaction in various everyday settings and strengthen their contribution to health are less well developed. Social support clearly reduces stress and the damage caused by psychological responses to it. Families and social networks influence patterns of living and general wellbeing, so initiatives should acknowledge, facilitate and further develop this care and support. The activities of health and social service agencies should help informal care givers to perform their tasks and increase their problem-solving capacities.

The main advantage of the settings approach to health promotion is that it allows the active involvement of the people most concerned and the tailoring of activities and initiatives to their specific requirements and local circumstances. Some examples are set out below.

Health-promoting schools   Schools are a key setting for the promotion of health. They can improve the health of the total school population and act as supportive environments for health. The social, environmental and ecological aspects of school life offer many opportunities to promote health both in the school and in the community outside. To implement this idea, a European network of schools is being set up jointly by WHO, the European Community and the Council of Europe. Its aim is to demonstrate that schools can provide a healthy and safe setting for working and learning. This can be achieved by addressing a number of different areas.

To start with, aims should be clearly set to promote health and safety for the whole school community, both pupils and adults, including support staff and teachers. Action can be taken in the physical school environment by improving buildings, play areas, facilities, safety measures and meals. A comprehensive health education curriculum should also be planned, which incorporates school health services.

The main aim of health education activities directed at pupils is that of empowerment. These activities should strive to enable all pupils to fulfil their full physical, psychological and social potential, to promote their self-esteem, and to equip them with the skills and knowledge necessary to make sound decisions about personal health. They should also help them to be active in the preservation and improvement of a safe physical environment, by becoming more aware as consumers. Efforts can be made to encourage healthy lifestyles, and to present a realistic and attractive range of healthy choices for schoolchildren and staff, as well as promoting individual, family and community responsibility for health. A further aim is to foster good relations between staff and pupils, among pupils, and among the school, home and community. Community resources to support health education and health promotion can be used to support these activities.

Health-promoting workplaces   The challenge here is to make employers understand that making the healthy choice is a wise business decision. This is equally true whether the employer is a local government authority, a university, a union or a hospital, or is in the commercial sector. In unhealthy working environments, many employees smoke, some are hypertensive, overweight and sedentary, some have mental health and substance abuse problems, many more are prone to lower back pain, and a large proportion experience burnout on the job.

The concept of the health-promoting company is inherently simple. Every owner, manager and employer, whether public or private, wants productivity. Satisfied workers contribute to the efficiency and effectiveness of the enterprise. Absenteeism is always costly. Unnecessary medical care costs are indefensible. Employees and their families are often important customers. It therefore follows that investment in the health of staff, through the creation of healthy workplaces, is a long-term benefit for the employing organization and the wider community as well as for individual employees. No country can afford to waste its health care resources, nor its labour force, nor the competitive economic viability of its commercial sector.

Healthy cities, healthy neighbourhoods, healthy homes   Significant experience has been gained through the WHO Healthy Cities project. This project demonstrates the importance of a strategy that balances a long-term sense of direction with the flexibility to take advantage of immediate opportunities for action. High visibility for local health issues is essential to gain the commitment of city politicians. Once such political commitment has been gained, departmental structures and managerial processes can be changed so that they allow wider participation in decisions that affect health. Innovative cooperative projects dealing with equity, housing, traffic control, recreation, access to public facilities and services, and other influences on the quality of city life then become possible.

Implementation depends on the strength of formal and informal mechanisms for intersectoral planning and decision-making. The links between political and executive leadership achieved through Healthy Cities coordinating committees and the interdepartmental communication that is generated can contribute greatly to success. The project offices linked to these committees provide neutral ground that facilitates coordination. They also offer leadership by exchanging information and advice and seeking out opportunities for action.

Especially important are mechanisms that enable interest groups, neighbourhood associations and individual citizens to take part in making plans and decisions about the settings in which they have a particular interest. In many Healthy Cities projects, citizen representatives are members of coordinating committees and neighbourhood associations are involved in defining the needs of the community. Community development and self-help activities are offered financial and other support. Experience in some local projects has shown how reaching vulnerable and disadvantaged groups through the settings of their daily lives can help them to articulate their views on priorities for action, empower them to work actively towards the promotion of health in a variety of ways, and facilitate their access to services.

Target 15 – Health competence

By the year 2000, accessible and effective education and training in health promotion should be available in all Member States, in order to improve public and professional competence in promoting health and increasing health awareness in other sectors.

This target can be achieved by:

- *making existing knowledge about health better known;*
- *emphasizing a wider range of lifestyle issues, including self-esteem, personal skills and social support;*
- *giving training and education in health promotion to all health professionals;*
- *training other groups and disciplines to increase awareness of health promotion opportunities;*
- *providing an effective infrastructure and adequate resources for implementing and coordinating health education programmes.*

Problem statement Health education programmes have been developing in Member States for over 25 years. In most cases, they have focused on giving individuals information that will help them change their behaviour in relation to specific risks to health. More recently, a number of programmes have addressed a wider range of lifestyle issues and emphasized the importance of self-esteem, personal skills, a sense of coherence in life and social support as prerequisites for healthy living. Despite this, lifestyles that are a risk to health continue to be widely prevalent as do unsupportive physical and social environments. Examples are smoking, problem drinking and harmful dietary practices, as well as environmental pollution and hazardous and stressful routines in the workplace.

Personal values, beliefs, social norms and cultural patterns are now widely recognized as major determinants of lifestyle. People's access to the prerequisites for health and the time to take advantage of them are equally important. Some people may damage their health because they are unaware of the risks they are taking or of the possible alternatives. Other people may be aware of the health risks. The daily influences exerted on them may nevertheless lead them into harmful eating, drinking and smoking habits, sedentary lifestyles with little time for physical activity and leisure, and stressful work routines. People who follow these patterns have little motivation to change their lives or to seek help. They lack the health competence and information that would enable them to make their own healthy choices and to resist negative social pressure. They are unable and unmotivated to take advantage of available help and to be effective advocates for the creation of healthy settings for living.

Problems can often be caused by a conflict between health education messages and messages that come from other, more compelling sources. Tobacco, alcohol and food advertisements often advocate unhealthy lifestyle practices but make the image very desirable. The advertisers have greater resources and better media expertise than are available to health educators. Health education needs to highlight the advantages and enjoyable aspects of health. The particular needs, concerns and living patterns of children, young people, women, older people, people with disabilities and ethnic minorities are not adequately reflected in educational programmes. New knowledge about physical activity, nutrition, stress, social support and other health issues takes a long time to reach the public. Confusion and loss of interest can result when this new knowledge is seen to contradict other, outdated information that is still being offered.

People need support and continuous encouragement when they decide to change their lifestyle patterns, but facilities and programmes to give assistance are not available in many communities. Most primary health care programmes do not treat disease prevention as a priority, nor do they incorporate effective health education. If health workers are to be effective advocates of health in the community, able to assist those seeking help, they need a better understanding of the effect of environmental factors on health, the influence of personal values and social norms on lifestyle choices, and the dynamics of motivation and behavioural change. Effective advocacy also requires health workers to be credible examples of healthy living, with their own lifestyles providing role models.

Budgetary resources, operational strategies and organizational structures are often inadequate to meet the challenge of a broader concept of health education. Current evidence of cost-effectiveness indicates that a much greater investment than the 1 – 3% of health budgets now allocated to health promotion will be needed if significant gains are to be achieved. In many Member States, health education authorities have not had strong enough mandates to provide effective visible leadership. Nor have they had sufficient autonomy to resist the political and social pressures that arise when lifestyle issues become controversial.

Effective health promotion requires approaches that actively involve leaders and workers in a variety of settings such as schools, workplaces, cities, labour unions, businesses and recreational centres. Unfortunately, the strategies often used are not comprehensive enough to enlist these resources and gain confidence and active support. Self-help groups concerned with health issues are also a valuable resource. But health authorities often do not recognize their efforts, do not provide financial and technical help to strengthen them, and do not explain adequately the problems of competing claims for resources. Advances are being made in the use of joint initiatives between the media and the community, such as community television, to build awareness and encourage discussion of environmental and similar issues. Much could be done to make more effective use of these approaches in health education. Of course, health education is not enough; a healthy choice needs to be available and easy in order to be made possible.

Suggested solutions The responsibility for health promotion is shared among individuals, community groups, health-related professions, health and social service institutions and governments. Health promotion supports personal and social development through a number of measures, among which health education plays a vital role *(1)*.

Within a health promotion framework, the central aim of health education should be to build health competence among the general population. This requires programmes to empower people, to improve their self-esteem and to help them develop and use their physical, mental and emotional capabilities to the fullest extent *(12)*. This can be achieved by strengthening their decision-making, interpersonal relationships and coping strategies, and emphasizing people's options so that they can exercise more control over their lives.

Health promotion must emphasize the economic, social and personal benefits of healthy living. It should adopt a positive approach that links health to environment, ecology and sustainable development. This means that health promotion is a key component of the health for all strategy, with health education its main tool. Health education messages need to be linked to other efforts to ensure people gain access to the prerequisites for health. For example, the impact of health education will be strengthened if it is visibly linked to pricing and taxation policies for tobacco, alcohol and food products. Health education can also contribute to the promotion of settings for healthy living. In the case of health-promoting schools, this means using opportunities throughout the curriculum to study and discuss all aspects of health. Support can also be given to the adult population, to become effective advocates for environmental improvement, linking health to ecological concerns and sustainable development.

Experience shows that effective national or federal health promotion institutes must have stronger mandates and a higher degree of autonomy. They can then provide leadership in developing strategy and mobilizing support at the community level, as well as providing technical and material resources, promoting research and disseminating new knowledge. These institutes should also develop educational courses and in-service training materials for all disciplines and professional groups. Training programmes for health promotion need to move from content input to competence output.

Strategies for health education must include a mix of centralized and decentralized actions, which recognize every setting in the community as an educational opportunity and investment (see target 14). For example, school and preschool health education, health promotion in the workplace and adult education can all contribute to physical fitness programmes. Self-help groups concerned with various disabilities or chronic diseases, as well as those for people wishing to stop smoking, control drinking or lose weight, are active in health education in many countries. Commercial organizations such as food suppliers are beginning to deliver health messages both at the workplace and in the marketplace. An important part of the strategy is to gain the confidence of such potential partners outside the health sector and to take the time to find ways of helping them achieve their own primary goals while delivering a health message. The emphasis needs to be on providing political, technical or financial support and on increasing awareness of health promotion opportunities among other groups and disciplines outside the health sector.

Health services should play a stronger role in promoting health and preventing disease by offering more health education (13). In primary health care, this will need innovative approaches to the organization of care, systems of remuneration and staffing arrangements (14). The basic and specialist training of physicians, nurses and other health professionals must give greater emphasis to health promotion. This means not only the inclusion of new subject matter that addresses social, economic and psychological factors in lifestyle choices, but also the use of different training methods.

Several major European educational campaigns for health offer new opportunities and support. Examples are the WHO Action Plan for a Tobacco-free Europe and the European Community programme, Europe Against Cancer.

The financial and economic constraints facing all Member States mean that the cost-effectiveness of health promotion – its value as an investment – must be clearly established if a sound investment policy is to be developed.

Target 16 – Healthy living

By the year 2000, there should be continuous efforts in all Member States to actively promote and support healthy patterns of living through balanced nutrition, appropriate physical activity, healthy sexuality, good stress management and other aspects of positive health behaviour.

This target can be achieved by taking a holistic approach to promoting healthy patterns of living, including:

* *increasing health and environmental awareness;*

* *developing and strengthening coping skills;*

* *promoting healthy eating patterns based on recommended nutrient standards and dietary guidelines;*

* *promoting healthy physical and other leisure activities;*

* *encouraging the giving and receiving of social support.*

Problem statement   Health promotion has refocused thinking about health to emphasize measures that help people to increase their wellbeing and protect against illness. These approaches have been described by using terms such as wellbeing, self-care, positive health behaviour and health maintenance. The continuing challenge for health promotion is to move beyond the focus on health-damaging behaviour that predominated in the past and to encourage examination of "the other side of the coin". It should emphasize health rather than disease and set up a continuum for action moving from prevention of disease to promotion of health. This is part of a wider change in values that is emerging in the Region, promoted by ecologists and environmental conservationists who are concerned about the future of the planet as well as its

people. Recognition of the interrelationship between health and the quality of the environment has introduced ecological ways of thinking into health promotion *(1)*.

Health promotion should take advantage of the growing body of knowledge about the positive effects on health of a range of personal skills, social factors and individual behaviours. Important among these are nutrition, physical activity, sexuality, stress management and family planning. Each of these areas poses its own particular problems to be overcome, if this target is to be achieved.

Nutrition   Overnutrition, undernutrition and unbalanced nutrition can all lead to health problems.

The percentage of total dietary energy from fat is a major indicator of a healthy diet. In 1989, much of the population of the Region lived in countries where the value of this indicator was considered too high (over 35%). Too little fibre and too much fat, sugar and salt in diets are common problems in many countries. Disorders associated with iodine deficiency are still endemic in parts of the Region. Problems are probably also caused by iron deficiency in women of reproductive age. Obesity is a significant problem in most countries and, since it is very difficult to cure when established, prevention is critical.

Places still exist in the Region where access to food is at times inadequate, raising questions of equity. In many countries undergoing transition from centralized economies, food shortages caused by problems in distribution and marketing periodically have serious consequences (6).

Poorly balanced nutrition may sometimes be due to lack of knowledge about diet, exacerbated by food advertising that encourages unhealthy choices. The menus in cafeterias, restaurants and fast-food outlets, however, have a more important effect on food choice. The development of food processing technology has influenced agricultural production and food availability more than any deliberate education campaign on nutrition. In many cases, however, the effects of technology have been beneficial. In developing healthy public policies, it is important to keep in mind that food processing is the largest industrial activity in some countries, exceeding by far that of alcohol and tobacco producers (15).

Physical activity   The contribution of physical fitness and appropriate physical activity to health and wellbeing has become widely acknowledged in many countries, but its full potential has yet to be realized. Physical fitness, acquired in youth and maintained throughout life by appropriate regular physical activity, helps maintain strength, allows the body to function in a healthy way, helps prevent disease and disability, and makes an important contribution to rehabilitation. Older people, in particular, should continue appropriate regular physical activity so as to preserve their functional capacity as long as possible. A challenge for health promotion in the future will be to disseminate knowledge about what constitutes appropriate physical exercise, counteracting any misleading claims from sections of the fitness industry. Another challenge will be to secure better access to sports and leisure facilities for all groups in the population.

Sexuality   Sexuality that involves supportive, caring, mutually consensual sexual relationships has a good effect on health. Conversely, a number of practices that are widely agreed to be undesirable have a deleterious effect on health. They include the sexual abuse of children; the physical, psychological and social exploitation of men and women through the purchase of their sexual services; unsafe sexual practices that lead to unwanted pregnancies; and sexual violence, often caused by alcohol and drug abuse.

Unresolved personal and social conflicts about acceptable expressions of sexuality can also be important contributors to individual health problems. People who hide their sexual orientation for fear of discrimination or other intolerant reactions, including physical violence, live less than fulfilling lives (16). They come under stress, experience alienation and social isolation, and can be placed in situations that are not conducive to safe sexual practices.

The emergence of the AIDS epidemic has increased the fear and conflict associated with issues of sexual behaviour. It has also led to the need for more open discussion, which in some countries is now taking place. Health promotion has an important role to play in these discussions, first, by highlighting the value of healthy sexuality as a contributor to health and, second, by supporting the adoption of safe sexual practices, which reduce the spread of HIV and other sexually transmitted diseases.

Stress management   The preservation of physical and mental health depends on people's ability to cope with the stresses of life, dealing with them in positive ways rather than through health-damaging behaviour *(12)*. Regular physical activity, relaxation and social interaction all promote health and are effective coping mechanisms. People who feel in control are less likely to become ill and, for them, stress can even have a positive effect. Unfortunately, the lives of many people do not allow balanced and controlled lifestyles that are conducive to health. Patterns of behaviour detrimental to health sometimes arise when individuals cannot cope adequately with stresses such as rapid social change, loneliness, bereavement, unemployment or unsatisfying work.

Family planning   All couples and individuals have the basic right to decide freely and responsibly the number and spacing of their children. In some places, this right is still not recognized and reproductive health choices still have to be made known and available. The lack of universal access

to safe and effective family planning can result in health problems, including psychological distress, raised abortion rates and unplanned pregnancies.

Suggested solutions   Healthy public policy *(2)* provides the foundation for achieving access to health through consumer products, living environments, and health and other services (see target 13). Efforts to achieve healthy settings for living in the city, at home, in the workplace and at school provide the strategy (see target 14). Health education is the process that creates the public awareness and support needed to maintain healthy settings and change lifestyles. The combination of policies and strategies needed varies according to the issues involved.

The introduction of ecological ways of thinking into health promotion, based on increasing awareness of the interrelationship between health and the quality of the environment, raises central questions for both research and action. It shifts the emphasis from the effect of individual behaviour on health to the influence of complex patterns of living. The changes in values promoted by ecologists and environmental conservationists need to be built on, and awareness of these interactions needs to be strengthened throughout the population.

Eating a balanced diet, engaging in regular physical activity, allowing time for rest and relaxation, and maintaining supportive social and sexual relationships all contribute to health. As understanding grows of what contributes to health, the close interaction between health and self-esteem, a sense of belonging and community, rewarding relationships and a strong sense of self-worth becomes clear. All these can be reinforced by actions taken to encourage the giving and receiving of social support.

Healthy nutrition In most societies, eating is an enjoyable experience associated with convivial social contact and the taste of good food. Scientific knowledge about nutrition has grown to the point where the contribution to health of various nutrients and amounts of food is reasonably well understood *(17)*. Personal taste, cultural traditions, patterns of social behaviour and the availability (including affordability) of food continue to be major determinants of what most people eat. Dietary guidelines have to be formulated in ways that make them useful and used. Measures that encourage the production of varied and nutritious food products and equitable access to good food should be a priority for policies on food supply and nutrition. The paper on a framework and options for action discussed at the first European Conference on Food and Nutrition Policy, in Budapest in 1990, provides a good starting point for such policies *(6)*.

Campaigns to promote healthy eating habits require the cooperation of food producers and retailers. In some cases, this will involve joint ventures in nutrition education, involving both the public and private sectors. The growing number of meals that people consume outside their homes means that institutional as well as private catering must be considered. Healthy nutrition will also be supported by action to improve food labelling (see targets 13 and 22) and associated measures to provide people with the necessary information and skills to become discerning consumers of food products. School health education and school meal services have an important role to play in encouraging healthy eating in future generations of adults. These educational programmes can be reinforced by complementary efforts in other settings such as the workplace and the home. In the broad attempt to help people with eating disorders, support for self-help groups is essential.

Adequate numbers of nutrition experts are needed to initiate many of the activities envisaged, and in many countries training such personnel will be an important priority.

Appropriate physical activity Appropriate physical activity can be a joyful experience and an important factor in improving the quality of life. Social attitudes towards physical activity have undergone a fundamental change over the past decade, providing an excellent basis for future action. Individuals should be encouraged to incorporate appropriate physical activity into their daily routine. This requires the promotion of sports and physical activity programmes, as well as action to make them more accessible to people in all social and age groups. Physical activities combined with recreation that strengthen social and family ties should be enjoyable and inexpensive. This requires town and country planning to protect both open countryside and parks for walking, relaxing and socializing and to provide opportunities for swimming and cycling. It should guarantee access to them for people with disabilities. Good health promotion campaigns stimulate awareness of activities that combine social involvement with physical activity. Dancing and other enjoyable forms of physical exercise are too often forgotten or not recognized as being healthy.

Healthy sexuality Sexuality is increasingly recognized as a strong human force that makes a positive contribution to health, when it is allowed expression in the context of caring, supportive, mutually consensual relationships. Member States should endorse the view that, in accordance with fundamental human rights, consenting adults can decide how to lead a healthy sexual life. Important differences in cultural values and traditions continue to exist between countries and in populations, but the rights of individuals to self-determination in their choice of sexual orientation must also be considered. The challenge for health promotion is to support positive expressions of sexuality in a manner sensitive to cultural values. This means taking action to support the rights of all adults to form sexual relationships with consenting partners of their own choice, and to promote respect and tolerance for individuals' decisions in this matter.

Knowledge about options, safe sexual practices and contraception is essential for healthy sexuality, which also requires individuals to have personal skills and characteristics such as self-esteem to enable them to define their wishes clearly. Sexual behaviour should be included as an integral part of school curricula on healthy living skills. Health promotion for adolescents and young adults should address sexuality and safe sexual practices. Condoms and other contraceptives should be easily available and affordable, to provide protection against sexually transmitted diseases, HIV infection and unwanted pregnancies. Counselling and other relevant services that are accessible, affordable and confidential should also be available to all population groups.

Action is also needed to combat the problems caused by unacceptable expressions of sexuality, such as the sexual abuse of children or adults and the exploitation of women and men who sell sex. In the long term, education for healthy sexuality along the lines set out above, together with other actions designed to achieve health for all, should reduce the occurrence of such expressions of sexuality. Where and when they do arise, a mix of appropriate legislative, educative

and administrative measures is required to deal with them. Relevant legislation will include protecting the rights of vulnerable groups such as children and women (see targets 7 and 8). The management of sexual abuse requires appropriate mechanisms to be available to health and social welfare agencies, which enable them to end the abuse in a manner that does not penalize the abused. For example, where abuse occurs in the home, the abused rather than the abuser is often removed from the home. Experience is growing in how best to deal with these problems. Services have been set up to help families and other social groups solve problems and resolve conflicts. Information for vulnerable groups, particularly children, should focus on ways of recognizing and exposing abuse and obtaining help. Special arrangements must be available to make the environments of vulnerable people safe, where necessary. In some countries, self-help groups and nongovernmental organizations have carried out innovative and effective activities in this area, which can provide examples for others.

Good stress management   Health promotion programmes must recognize the primary importance of coping ability as a factor in lifestyle choices. Overeating, smoking, drinking, drug taking and lack of physical exercise are indications of an inability to cope with stress.

Health professionals need to develop an interest and skills in health promotion and be ready to study the effectiveness of new approaches. Active methods of stress management that enhance health must be devised and promoted. These can include problem-solving skills, a proper balance between work and leisure, the ability to relax in stressful situations, and the use of sports, meditation and other recreational activities. The emphasis should be on empowering people with the necessary skills to cope effectively with stress, as well as trying to remove the causes of stress (see targets 1, 2, 14).

Coping ability can be strengthened by measures to promote settings that support healthy patterns of living. These are settings that encourage social interaction, recognize and facilitate systems of informal social support, allocate time for leisure and relaxation, and encourage appropriate physical activity. They take a variety of forms. In the home setting, whether in a rural or urban area, opportunities should exist for social contact and recreation, and the settlement design should allow space for recreation and encourage a strong sense of community. Workplaces must be designed to recognize the importance of social contacts between workers. Health-promoting schools need to incorporate health throughout the curriculum, provide opportunities for physical activity and for the reinforcement of healthy behaviour, and introduce programmes to strengthen coping skills in students *(4)*. Communities also need to provide programmes on stress management that are particularly attuned to at-risk population groups such as unemployed people, migrants or refugees.

Family planning Measures to support family planning must recognize people's right to decide the number and spacing of their children. This right must be supported by universal access to safe and effective means of contraception, counselling on reproductive choices, and services such as the termination of pregnancy where appropriate and legal. This will require additional government support in many Member States.

School health education has an important role to play in promoting healthy sexuality as a basis for individual and family life. Such education must encourage men and women to accept equal responsibility for the avoidance of unwanted pregnancies, for family planning and for child rearing. Social policies should facilitate this more equal division of responsibility in family planning and child rearing, and include an emphasis on communicating the opportunities for men in these roles.

Target 17 – Tobacco, alcohol and psychoactive drugs

By the year 2000, the health-damaging consumption of dependence-producing substances such as alcohol, tobacco and psychoactive drugs should have been significantly reduced in all Member States.

This target can be achieved if well balanced policies and programmes in regard to the consumption and production of these substances are implemented at all levels and in different sectors to:

- *increase the number of nonsmokers to at least 80% of the population and protect nonsmokers from involuntary exposure to tobacco smoke;*

- *reduce alcohol consumption by 25%, with particular attention to reducing harmful use;*

- *obtain a sustained and continuing reduction in the abuse of psychoactive drugs, including inappropriate use of prescribed drugs.*

Problem statement   Behaviour that is a risk to health has been a preoccupation of health education for several decades. The use of tobacco, alcohol and both illegal and prescribed psychoactive drugs have received the most attention. Patterns of consumption in each of these three areas vary throughout Member States, but trends toward greater use are still found in many places. In terms of tobacco consumption, 68% of the total population of the Region live in countries where consumption levels are not yet decreasing, while 61% of the total population of the Region live in countries where alcohol consumption levels are increasing.

Tobacco and alcohol use are part of the daily lives of many people in the Region. Attitudes towards the use of different substances vary in fundamental ways, and there are significant differences between parts of the Region. The drinking of alcohol is widely accepted in almost every country. Smoking is becoming socially less acceptable, especially in western and northern Europe, following persistent health education on this issue. While the consumption of illegal drugs has been increasing for several years, this problem has not yet received widespread public attention.

Differences in consumption patterns and trends between groups in the population pose serious problems for the development of preventive measures. Tobacco consumption, for example, is growing in some places among younger age groups and women. The most serious concerns about drug use also focus on the young. At the same time, substance abuse in general is growing among people who have fewer economic and social opportunities, raising questions of equity in health.

Effective policies require an appropriate balance between three different control measures. Education and support, legislation and regulations, and fiscal policies all have a role. Policy development must ensure that the health impact of fiscal policies is not neglected. Governments must combat misleading accusations that policies that aim to reduce consumption inhibit individual freedom of choice.

Tobacco   Smoking is now recognized as a major cause of lung cancer, ischaemic heart disease, chronic bronchitis and emphysema. Concern is also growing about low birth weight in infants whose mothers smoked during pregnancy, and the development of cancer and other diseases among nonsmokers who are exposed to tobacco smoke. During 1985, an estimated total of just over 1.1 million deaths in the European Region were due to tobacco *(18)*. During 1990, the figure was just over 1.2 million. In 1995, it is expected to be be nearly 1.4 million.

The general pattern of smoking in the Region has changed considerably over the last 30 years. Significant improvements have been achieved in countries that have introduced comprehensive tobacco control policies and well developed education programmes. While consumption has decreased in the Region as a whole, it has continued to increase in some countries. Women and young people are now the targets of the most aggressive marketing strategies of the tobacco industry. Major cigarette producers are also taking advantage of the new marketing opportunities in the central and eastern parts of the Region.

The harmful effects of tobacco use, in both economic and social terms, are now widely recognized. Nevertheless, the large profits and perceived economic advantages associated with the production and marketing of tobacco have severely limited the policy options for reducing consumption. Some governments neglect the potential health impact of fiscal policies.

Alcohol Drinking alcohol is a common feature of the cultures of the European Region. It is associated with conviviality, consumption of food and relief of stress, and its widespread acceptance has a fundamental influence on alcohol policy in most Member States.

The likelihood of health problems developing in association with alcohol use increases as the consumption of alcohol increases. Most health-related problems occur in association with habitual drinking in excess of appropriate levels (which depend on sex and other factors such as body weight). Other health problems arise when the concentrated consumption of large amounts of alcohol in a short period of time ("binge drinking") results in violence or road traffic accidents.

In view of this, the general increase in the rates of alcohol consumption in most countries of the Region from the mid-1950s to about 1980 is disturbing. Consumption doubled in some countries and trebled in a few. The most recent trends for the period 1986 – 1989 show that increases have continued in countries covering 61% of the total population of the Region. Trends have been markedly different for the consumption of beer, wines and spirits. Wine and beer have been substituted for spirits in some places, beer for wine in others, and wine for beer elsewhere. There are only two countries in the Region (covering only some 3% of the regional population) in which the consumption of spirits, wines *and* beer decreased between 1986 and 1989. The number of occasions on which it is considered appropriate to use alcohol has also tended to increase, while drinking has spread among groups where it was formerly less prevalent, such as women and young people. The introduction and acceptance in some countries of low alcohol beer has been a welcome development.

Psychoactive drugs The use of illegal drugs has become more common in many countries in the Region over the last two decades. The harmful effects on individuals, their families and society in general are now widely recognized. While some countries show an encouraging trend towards the levelling off of drug use, prevalence continues to increase in others. About one million people in the Region are currently estimated to be dependent on illegal drugs. As economic and social changes occur in the central and eastern part of the Region, fear is growing that trafficking in illegal drugs will become more common. The spread of AIDS and HIV infection has added a serious new dimension to the illegal drug problem and is a cause for increased social concern. The situation is exacerbated by the ineffectiveness of drug control policies, by insufficient coordination of drug control programmes both in and between countries, and by the ineffectiveness of programmes aimed at prevention, treatment and rehabilitation.

Awareness is also growing of the harmful consequences of using prescribed psychoactive drugs, owing to both inappropriate prescribing and the growth of an illicit market. It is, unfortunately, still common practice to turn to drugs to deal with social and psychological problems. The overprescribing of psychoactive drugs, especially to women and elderly people, is a serious aspect of this problem. In some countries in the Region, the problems are compounded by the ineffective enforcement of laws controlling prescription.

Suggested solutions Measures to prevent smoking and the harmful use of alcohol and drugs are an important aspect of healthy public policy (see target 13). Because of the degree of social concern and conflict associated with the use of these substances and the economic and political interests involved, strategies in this area should be based on clear policies with achievable objectives. An appropriate balance should be attained between educational and regulatory measures, to reflect political and cultural norms.

International collaboration is crucial in controlling the harmful use of substances. A good example of such collaboration is control on trafficking in illegal drugs carried out through the United Nations Commission on Narcotics. The influence of European Community measures on the production and marketing of alcohol and tobacco, including subsidies for production in both areas, suggests a role for public health advocacy in these areas. The international marketing practices adopted by tobacco and alcohol companies require equivalent cooperation at the international level to combat them, as is provided in the WHO Action Plan for a Tobacco-free Europe. A European Alcohol Action Plan has been prepared.

Clear leadership at the highest appropriate level in each country is necessary to prevent the harm caused by substance use. This must be supported by strategies for local action that involve the creation of settings for healthy living and the use of health education, especially in schools and at the workplace. The design of health education programmes must be in line with the model of health education discussed earlier. They must recognize the importance of economic and social constraints on the individual choice of behaviour. They must recognize that behaviour damaging to health may be adopted as a means to cope with daily stress. Treatment and rehabilitation programmes should be designed to support and complement the work of self-help groups and nongovernmental organizations.

Tobacco At the European Conference on Tobacco Policy in Madrid in 1988, Member States agreed to promote nonsmoking and smoke-free environments as the norm in the Region. This can be achieved through a combination of educational programmes, regulatory measures (including taxation, pricing and controls on advertising), environmental controls creating smoke-free environments, and programmes to support people who wish to stop smoking. The challenge for the next decade is to implement the measures adopted in the guidelines that came from the Conference.

The WHO publication that resulted from the Conference *(5)* sets out guidelines that include a charter against tobacco, ten strategies for a smoke-free Europe and a check-list of over 100 activities to be pursued by countries throughout the Region. The charter promotes the rights of all people to be protected from tobacco smoke and tobacco promotion, to be informed of the unparalleled risks of tobacco use, and to breathe air free from tobacco smoke at work, on public transport and in public places, and the rights of smokers to receive help and encouragement to overcome their addiction to tobacco.

These rights can be fulfilled by governments, businesses, public services, regional and local health services, and nongovernmental organizations across the Region. Relevant action includes legislation and fiscal measures to raise the price and curtail the production and consumption of tobacco, to free people from the promotion of tobacco, and to provide comprehensive educational programmes for children and adults to help them live free from addiction to tobacco. The suggested actions gain particular strength from the many alliances being built to counter pressures to sell tobacco to young people.

Policies that have achieved the most significant results are comprehensive in their approach. They include, for example, reducing the availability of tobacco to children, providing intensive health education in schools, imposing strong controls on advertising, running vigorous anti-tobacco campaigns, making provisions for smoke-free public places, and maintaining relatively high prices through taxation. Where a taxation policy is used, prices should keep pace with or exceed inflation.

Health education appears to be most successful when carried out as part of the school and preschool health curriculum and in work settings. An important development in recent years has been a steady increase in the number of settings that are established as smoke-free environments. They include public places, transport facilities, worksites, hospitals and clinics. More emphasis needs to be put on health promotion in schools, preschool settings and the workplace, on smoking cessation, and on programmes for expectant young parents. Financing will have to be assured for these activities.

Some Member States are concerned that measures to discourage tobacco growing and cigarette manufacture will have adverse effects on the economy and on employment, at least in the short term. More careful analysis is needed, both in countries and at the international level, of the economic consequences of tobacco production. More health-oriented goods that can replace tobacco need to be identified, and strategies developed to compensate for lost tax revenue.

Alcohol The health and social problems caused by alcohol use can be prevented or reduced both by general measures to reduce alcohol consumption and by specific measures aimed at high-risk groups and situations.

An effective alcohol policy must tackle both supply, through controls on production, distribution, advertising and price, and demand, through health education and prevention programmes. In addition, it must include comprehensive treatment services. The relative importance of these instruments will vary from one country to another. Countries that have few controls on the supply side tend to emphasize treatment or health education and prevention. Control policies have been shown to reduce levels of alcohol consumption and thereby the magnitude of alcohol-related problems. Political acceptability and public support are vital to the effectiveness and continuity of an alcohol policy. In countries where restrictive policies have been introduced without sufficient public support, an increase in illicit production has followed.

The alcohol, catering and entertainment industries are major employers and contributors to gross domestic product and tax revenue. The industries' structure is such that a small number of firms control most of the market. This, together with the industries' international organizations, should allow negotiation of a common approach towards a code of practice on self-regulation, for a product that causes society not only harm but also some benefit.

At the local level, broad-based multisectoral community programmes are needed to achieve community-wide changes in lifestyle and reduce the sale and use of alcohol. Individual motivation and ability to avoid the harm done by alcohol use can be strengthened in the settings of everyday life such as health-promoting schools, health-promoting workplaces and healthy cities (see target 14).

Educational campaigns not only have an impact on individual drinkers, but also raise support for programmes that urge moderation in the sale and use of alcohol. The theme and message of such campaigns should be to drink less often and less on each occasion.

Primary health care is the setting where individuals at risk from heavy drinking can be identified and helped to reduce their alcohol consumption. Instruments are available for screening and intervention in this setting. A number of innovative approaches to the treatment of people who drink too much have been successful and should be more widely disseminated.

Psychoactive drugs   Better information material and programmes are needed for use in schools, workplaces and the mass media. An important aim is to help people understand the influence of social and cultural attitudes on the use of drugs and other substances as a means of coping. More effective mechanisms of social support should be developed for those who are especially vulnerable to substance abuse. These mechanisms could include a broad range of outreach activities, self-help groups, treatment centres, half-way houses and shelters, all aimed at improving prevention, treatment and rehabilitation services for people with drug and alcohol problems, including social violence. More vigorous research is needed to develop innovative approaches to prevention, taking into consideration a broad range of possible measures in different sectors. Early recognition and intervention at the primary health care level are especially important. Similarly, the development of better methods for evaluating treatment programmes and a systematic search for more effective methods of treatment must be given high priority.

Inappropriate prescribing of psychoactive drugs has harmful consequences. Coordinated action is needed to increase the emphasis on appropriate prescribing practices in the training of health professionals. Such training needs to encourage the use of other, more appropriate therapeutic measures instead. Various alternatives exist for combating the depression or anxiety caused by what are, at root, social rather than psychological problems. These alternatives include self-help groups, and groups and courses facilitated by experts. Training and education in health promotion for all health professionals, as discussed in target 15, will help to increase their awareness of these alternatives.

References

1. Ottawa Charter for Health Promotion. *Health promotion*, **1**(4): iii – v (1986).
2. The Adelaide recommendations: healthy public policy. *Health promotion*, **3**(2): 183 – 186 (1988).
3. *Sundsvall statement on supportive environments for health*. Third International Conference on Health Promotion. Geneva, World Health Organization, 1992 (document WHO/HED/92.1).
4. *Approaches to stress management in the community setting*: report on a WHO Consultation. Copenhagen, WHO Regional Office for Europe, 1992 (document EUR/ICP/PSF 028).
5. *It can be done. A smoke-free Europe*. Copenhagen, WHO Regional Office for Europe, 1990 (WHO Regional Publications, European Series, No. 30).
6. *Food and nutrition policy in Europe*: report on a WHO Conference. Copenhagen, WHO Regional Office for Europe, 1991 (document EUR/ICP/NUT 133).
7. JOOSSENS, L. & RAW, M. Tobacco and the European common agricultural policy. *British journal of addiction*, **86**: 1191 – 1202 (1991).
8. ROBERTS, J.L. *Code busting by tobacco companies*. Project Smokefree, North Western Regional Health Authority, England, 1987.
9. KICKBUSCH, I. ET AL. Healthy public policy: a strategy to implement the health for all philosophy at various governmental levels. *In*: Evers, A. et al., ed. *Healthy public policy at the local level*. Frankfurt/New York, Campus/Westview, 1989, pp. 1 – 6.
10. *Investment in health. Proceedings of the International Conference on Health Promotion, Bonn, 17 – 19 December 1990*. Bonn, Wissenschaftliches Institut der Ärzte Deutschlands, 1990 (document EUR 14281 EN).
11. *Environment and health. The European Charter and commentary*. Copenhagen, WHO Regional Office for Europe, 1990 (WHO Regional Publications, European Series, No. 35).
12. BOSMA, M.W.M., ED. *Mental health promotion and prevention in schools*. Utrecht, Dutch Centre for Health Education and Health Promotion, 1991.
13. *Prevention of mental, psychosocial and neurological disorders in the European Region*. Copenhagen, WHO Regional Office for Europe, 1991 (document EUR/PSF/88.1).
14. *Psychosocial interventions in primary health care settings in Europe*: report on a WHO Consultation. Copenhagen, WHO Regional Office for Europe, 1991 (document EUR/ICP/PSF 020).
15. *Food and health data. Their use in nutrition policy-making*. Copenhagen, WHO Regional Office for Europe, 1991 (WHO Regional Publications, European Series, No. 34).
16. SKETCHLEY, J.M. *Psychosexual services in selected European countries*: report on a WHO Study. Copenhagen, WHO Regional Office for Europe, 1991 (document EUR/ICP/MCH 523).

17. JAMES, W.P.T. *Healthy nutrition. Preventing nutrition-related diseases in Europe.* Copenhagen, WHO Regional Office for Europe, 1988 (WHO Regional Publications, European Series, No. 24).

18. PETO, R. ET AL. Mortality from tobacco in developed countries: indirect estimation from national vital statistics. *Lancet*, **339**: 1268 – 1278 (1992).

5

Healthy environment

Targets 18 – 25 are concerned with the contribution of the environment to health and are based on the strategies of the European Charter on Environment and Health. They link together the emerging commitment to environmental policies that could lead to ecologically sustainable development, the prevention and control of risks to the population, and equitable access to healthy environments. Their aim is to provide people with opportunities to live in communities with socially and physically supportive environments (see Fig. 4).

Since the United Nations conference in Rio de Janeiro in 1992, the consensus has been that the highest priority needs to be given to protecting the environment. Global policy aims at development that is balanced and sustainable, so that socio-economic growth and the ecosystem are in harmony and mutually supportive. Highly industrialized Europe has a particular responsibility in the global community.

Europe is far from the ideal of an environment that is free from hazards to health, provides psychological and aesthetic support for personal development and is equitably accessible to all. An important Region-wide consensus, based on a strong concern with health issues, led to the unanimous adoption of the European Charter on Environment and Health *(1)* by 29 Member States and the Commission of the European Communities in 1989, as a set of principles to guide the development of national policies. The 1991 Sundsvall Conference on supportive environments for health showed that there is considerable interaction between the physical and social environments *(2)*.

The health of the environment The environment has gradually improved in several countries, especially in the north of Europe. Air quality has improved owing to reductions in sulfur dioxide emission and the lead content of petrol. Many countries have also achieved improvements in areas such as housing, parks, nuclear safety and the social environment. On a regional scale, however, the overall environment has not improved in the last decades owing to growing industrialization, the introduction of new technologies, the increasing use of chemicals, more intensive agricultural

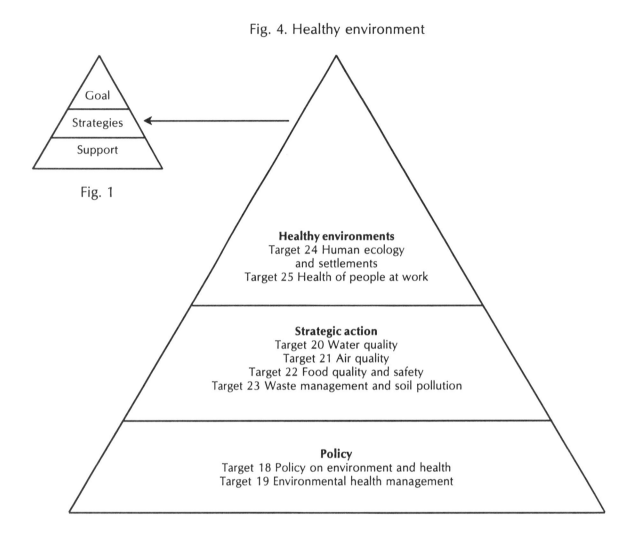

Fig. 4. Healthy environment

Fig. 1

Goal
Strategies
Support

Healthy environments
Target 24 Human ecology
and settlements
Target 25 Health of people at work

Strategic action
Target 20 Water quality
Target 21 Air quality
Target 22 Food quality and safety
Target 23 Waste management and soil pollution

Policy
Target 18 Policy on environment and health
Target 19 Environmental health management

practices, increasing energy consumption, the growing consumption of material goods in general, growing amounts of industrial and community waste, increasing motor vehicle traffic and rapid urbanization. In many countries, air pollution, exposure to chemicals, the contamination of soil and water, hazards to food safety and exposure to biological agents have tended to increase.

For a multitude of reasons, the state of the environment varies widely within the Region. By the 1970s and 1980s, the northern and western parts had established infrastructures and policies for environment and health. They are now dealing with the complex environmental problems of post-industrial society. Elsewhere, particularly in eastern, central and southern parts of the Region, basic problems of community hygiene and sanitation remain. Unchecked industrial pollution in several central and eastern European countries is of particular concern.

Environment-related health problems

In post-industrial societies, the major environment-related diseases and disorders include cancer, cardiovascular diseases, respiratory disorders, allergies, reproductive problems, locomotor disorders, psychological and neurological disorders, and accidental injuries. Since large groups of the population are exposed to many risk factors, even a small increase in risk levels may significantly increase the incidence of a particular disorder.

The environment is usually only one of several causal factors in disease development, and it interacts with biological agents, lifestyles and hereditary factors. Its relative importance is rarely known with any precision. In some cases, different factors are synergistic and multiply the risk from the individual factors. Despite scientific uncertainties, a reasonable conclusion is that an improvement in the environment is likely to increase health and reduce illness. No evidence exists of any health benefits from poor environments.

In countries with less developed infrastructures, the traditional epidemic diseases, often of microbiological origin, may still pose important problems. They are associated with environmental deficiencies (for example, enteric diseases in children are due to poor sanitation) and with low water and food hygiene. Similarly, certain occupational activities may result in specific diseases such as pneumoconiosis. Achieving reductions in these environment-related diseases does not primarily require new knowledge and technology, but better management. The most difficult environmental problems come together in the urban environment, which requires particular attention.

Emphasis on implementation

Current work on the environment and health shows that stress put on the environment soon results in changes that are an impending hazard to human health. Preventive measures should therefore be aimed at areas such as air, water, soil, waste and food, as well as specific living and working environments.

Every Member State should formulate and implement an effective policy for environment and health, taking into account the best principles of disease prevention, health promotion and human ecology. Implementation requires well integrated planning and managerial systems at all levels and a clear identification of priorities. No practical activity can be carried out without well functioning infrastructures and adequate human resources and equipment. Particular attention should be given to the mechanisms that ensure multisectoral collaboration in practice. In certain parts of the Region, improvements in the basic infrastructures of environmental hygiene are also needed.

Environmental problems cross national borders, so active collaboration is needed between countries and with international organizations. This should facilitate the transfer of scientific knowledge, experience and technology, and should benefit from the expanding activities of the WHO Regional Office for Europe through its Centre for Environment and Health.

Better national and international information systems on environment and health are needed to improve the awareness, motivation and participation of the public, politicians and industry. International collaboration is also required to help some countries improve their infrastructures, training and access to resources.

Target 18 – Policy on environment and health

By the year 2000, all Member States should have developed, and be implementing, policies on the environment and health that ensure ecologically sustainable development, effective prevention and control of environmental health risks and equitable access to healthy environments.

This target can be achieved if all Member States adhere to the principles of the Frankfurt Charter and collaborate internationally in the control of transfrontier and global environmental threats. This will require action in all Member States to:

- *review, adapt and develop their environment and health policies in the light of the European Charter on Environment and Health, as an essential component of health for all policy;*

- *formulate and implement country, regional and/or local laws, regulations, incentives and practices accordingly;*

- *establish country, regional and local mechanisms for involving people in policy development and implementation.*

Problem statement Today, people are well aware that the general environment is deteriorating. Human health is influenced both by threats to animal and plant life, and by constraints on economic development in large parts of the planet. The environment itself can have both positive and negative effects on health. The agents involved can be the places where people live, work or relax, specific agents such as microorganisms, physical forces or chemicals, or more general agents such as the atmosphere, soil and water.

Until a few years ago, health policies had rarely been linked to concerns with the general environment and so had not benefited from the strong popular ecological movement. While collaboration in the prevention and control of health risks in the environment has been improving, there is still scope for further intersectoral action between sectors, levels, institutions and countries.

A common aim for the general environment, as well as health, is an ecologically sustainable development brought about by the prudent management of the earth's resources and the biosphere, without jeopardizing future generations. The European Region may be failing to achieve sustainability. Evidence for this is the depletion of the stratospheric ozone layer, the deterioration of large areas of the Mediterranean and Baltic seas and Europe's major rivers, reliance on energy from high sulfur fossil fuels that increase acid deposition and groundwater pollution, the wide use of grossly polluting technology, ill-considered land use and agricultural practices, and general profligacy and carelessness with resources and waste products.

Many problems in the past resulted from the false notion that the needs of the environment and health conflicted with those of economic development.

Some sections of the population are especially vulnerable. People who work with certain processes or live near certain industrial plants may be particularly exposed to specific agents. Infants and children take in more of a contaminant relative to their size than do adults. Social equity in terms of access to a healthy environment has not been achieved, nor has it entered fully into the public awareness.

The interaction of the physical environment with the social environment and people's lifestyles has many effects on health. In some countries, however, environment and health policies are still sometimes confined to inspectorate functions in the physical environment.

Suggested solutions
The governments of the Region and the Commission of the European Communities have acknowledged the growing concern for the environment. They recognized the urgency of effective action to protect the environment and health by unanimously adopting the European Charter on Environment and Health in December 1989.

The principles of the Charter provide a framework, linked to the health for all strategy, from which Member States can derive policies for environment and health. The Charter emphasizes predictive and preventive strategies, the need to reverse negative trends in the environment, and the use of the environment as a resource for improving living conditions and increasing wellbeing.

The Charter also proposes the entitlements and responsibilities of individuals and of public and private organizations, the principles of public policy, its strategic elements and the priorities for prevention. It suggests arrangements for the management and control of environmental health hazards and provides guidance for future activities. The practical implementation of its principles is particularly stressed *(1)*.

In the European Region, important concerns about the environment include: global disturbances such as the destruction of the ozone layer and climatic change; urban development, planning and renewal to protect health and promote wellbeing; safe and adequate drinking-water supplies and hygienic waste disposal for all urban and rural communities; the quality of surface, ground and coastal waters; the microbiological and chemical safety of food; the environmental and health impact of various energy options, of transport (especially road transport) and agricultural practices, including the use of fertilizers and pesticides, and of waste disposal; air quality, especially in relation to oxides of sulfur and nitrogen, photochemical oxidants and volatile organic compounds; indoor air quality (residential, recreational and occupational) including the effects of radon, exposure to tobacco smoke, chemicals and biological contaminants; persistent chemicals and those having chronic effects; hazardous wastes including their management, transport and disposal; biotechnology and, in particular, genetically modified organisms; contingency planning for and in response to accidents and disasters; and cleaner technologies as preventive measures. Their priority will differ from country to country.

Where possible, a preventive approach should be adopted in tackling these priorities. This includes protecting the health of vulnerable groups. Careful risk and environmental impact assessments should be undertaken before any new technologies, industrial sites or chemicals are introduced.

A multisectoral approach is necessary, and all involved – governments, communities, industry and individuals – must assume greater responsibility and accountability. This will, in many countries, require a review and adjustment of national and local laws, regulations, incentives and practices. For example, the principle that the polluter pays should be adopted. This means that every public and private body that causes or may cause damage to the environment is made financially responsible.

The Charter calls for effective monitoring, analysis and assessment of environmental health hazards, as well as appropriate research on preventive technologies and environmental epidemiology. All this would be aided by the collection, analysis and assessment of data on environment and health at the national level in the Region. If governments communicated such information to responsible authorities, communities and individuals, as well as to those making decisions on environment and health, this would have a crucial effect on the implementation of environment and health policies and on the shaping of public opinion.

The WHO Healthy Cities project has demonstrated that great benefits are derived from linking social environment policies with the promotion of healthy lifestyles. This link aims to ensure that the environment not only is free from health hazards but also provides a supportive basis for healthy living by all people.

Since the adoption of the Charter, Member States have been reviewing and strengthening their policies to meet the environment and health problems of the 1990s and to reverse the current declining trends in the quality of the environment. Some governments have already published countrywide policy documents for the environment, which include aspects relevant to health and outline strategies for environment and health for the year 2000 and beyond. These policies should not only tackle newly emerging environmental health hazards and risks, but also prevent the perpetuation of established health hazards and risks in the environment.

The European Region should also contribute to international programmes for the control of global environmental threats. All the countries in the Region should therefore support the implementation of international agreements on the control of environmental threats, such as the Montreal Protocol on Substances that Deplete the Ozone Layer, the Basel Convention on the Control of Transboundary Movements of Hazardous Wastes and their Disposal, and the United Nations Economic Commission for Europe's Convention on Long-range Transboundary Air Pollution. They should also collaborate in subregional programmes such as the United Nations Environment Programme's Mediterranean Action Plan and the Helsinki Convention to protect the Baltic Sea.

Target 19 – Environmental health management

By the year 2000, there should be effective management systems and resources in all Member States for putting policies on environment and health into practice.

This target can be achieved by implementing the policies advocated in target 18 following the strategic elements and priorities of the Frankfurt Charter. This requires action to conserve natural resources, promote sustainable development, control health risks in air, water, soil, food and waste, and create environments that support health and wellbeing where people live and work. It can be brought about if Member States:

- *establish systems for environmental monitoring and impact assessment, linking environment and health information;*

- *use country, regional and local mechanisms to involve government, industry, primary producers and community groups in environmental health action based on full sharing of information;*

- *consider the impact on environment and health of policies and strategies in sectors such as urban planning, energy, transport, industrial development and agriculture;*

- *mobilize adequate resources from all sectors to achieve environmental health targets;*

- *develop management systems, operational methods, appropriate technology, research and training to support environmental health management.*

Problem statement   Managing the environment has become a high political priority, owing to the significant impact on human health of technological accidents involving chemicals and radioactivity. Current political, economic and social change in the Region has further raised awareness and public anxiety about such incidents.

Significant progress has been made in the development of legal frameworks that permit the introduction of standards for acceptable levels of hazardous chemicals in food, air and drinking-water. Particular efforts have been made to harmonize the implementation of environmental standards throughout the countries of the European Community. Usually, however, monitoring and control strategies tend to be limited to single sources of exposure and focus on a dozen or so of the most incriminated substances. Moreover, many of the strategies are based on compliance with standards that are not always directly related to actual exposure. Some countries in the Region do, however, practise an integrated pollution control policy.

Although specific hazards to health in the environment must be identified and controlled, it is their total impact and their interaction with social conditions and lifestyles that are important.

In some countries, the responsibility for different media (such as air, water or food) is split between a multitude of institutions, levels and sectors. This makes it difficult to take a coherent and comprehensive management approach, or even to collect and link information on exposure and risk. Despite differences in the organization of environmental health services between countries, most are geared to the control of environmental health hazards rather than their prevention.

A number of countries lack an adequate infrastructure and mechanisms to anticipate intentional or unintentional releases of toxic chemicals and other hazards and to assess the extent of damage caused. They are also ill-equipped to estimate the contribution of environmental and other factors to local and national health status. In many countries, the tendency is to focus on isolated events and problems, rather than to take an epidemiological view. This weakness in information systems means that no indicators of impact and quality have been developed, so it is difficult to monitor the effectiveness of policies and strategies.

The inadequacy of public information and health education has inhibited public involvement in environmental health management. Priorities have sometimes been set on the basis of emotions and pressure from interest groups, rather than of scientific facts.

The numbers and qualification of environmental health personnel have increased to an appropriate level in most European countries. There may, however, be too few experienced personnel in the central

and eastern parts of the Region to cope with the accumulated problems of industrial pollution.

Suggested solutions   The European Charter on Environment and Health provides the policy framework and strategy for environment and health in the Region (see target 18). The aim is not merely a low level of health hazards, but a clean and harmonious environment that supports health and stimulates healthy lifestyles. The emphasis is on strategies that are collaborative, predictive and preventive and are properly planned, implemented and evaluated.

The health sector has a leading role in the epidemiological surveillance and assessment of the health impact of environmental factors and in communicating conclusions to other sectors of society and the general public.

A comprehensive strategy for prevention requires appropriate incentives, technologies, and legislative and administrative mechanisms. It also needs to ensure that information about the importance of prevention reaches all sections of the community. Fiscal, administrative and economic instruments and land-use planning all have an important role in promoting environmental conditions conducive to health.

Managing the implementation of shared environment and health objectives requires activities, resources and support from different levels, sectors and public and private institutions. They have distinct but complementary roles and responsibilities in the development of health criteria and indicators for evaluation, in the strengthening of environmental health services, and in the creation of durable intersectoral links.

Priorities and standards that are set on the basis of scientific risk assessment can make a useful contribution to feasible, timely and cost-effective action. The Charter specifically refers to the WHO guidelines for drinking-water quality (3) and the WHO air quality guidelines for Europe (4).

As for strategies for the control of chemicals, they should include notification procedures for new chemicals and systematic examination of existing chemicals. Contingency planning is vital and should deal with all types of serious accident, including those with transfrontier consequences.

The needs of the countries in the central and eastern part of the Region differ widely between countries and areas. But they all present a new challenge for the development of appropriate, coordinated control and monitoring strategies. Support and expertise from other countries in the Region may be needed. The first priority is to reduce the known health hazards in the environment and to reverse the environmental decay and neglect as part of economic reconstruction.

Medical and other professionals, such as toxicologists and epidemiologists, should pay greater attention to the environment. National and international programmes of training in such disciplines should be strengthened accordingly. Similarly,

greater emphasis should be put on the health aspects of environmental impact assessment. Research programmes in environmental epidemiology should be encouraged at all levels and should aim to clarify the links between the environment and health. Collaborative international studies in toxicology and epidemiology could play an important role.

Action in the environment and health field requires data of good and comparable quality. The development of environmental health data and information systems based on environmental epidemiology should therefore be encouraged. Strategies for preventing noncommunicable diseases, in particular, would benefit from better prediction, identification, monitoring and assessment of the impact of the environment on health.

A good share of the practical implementation of environment and health strategies takes place at the local level. The role of communities, interest groups and individuals is crucial, and better mechanisms are needed to assist their participation. People should be given a clear voice in decisions about their own environment and health, not only because they have a right to know but also because active communication and participation motivate people to protect the environment and to use it as a resource for health.

Target 20 – Water quality

By the year 2000, all people should have access to adequate supplies of safe drinking-water and the pollution of groundwater sources, rivers, lakes and seas should no longer pose a threat to health.

This target can be achieved if water conservation strategies are implemented to meet evolving environmental health problems and needs. Achievement of these strategies requires:

- *providing access to adequate and continuous supplies of safe drinking-water that meet WHO drinking-water quality guidelines;*

- *ensuring effective wastewater disposal, sanitation and protection of drinking-water resources;*

- *taking appropriate intersectoral action to prevent contamination of water sources by agricultural and industrial pollution.*

Problem statement   During the International Drinking Water Supply and Sanitation Decade, almost all settlements in the Region were connected to a supply of drinking-water. On the whole, urban areas are well off, though some slum districts in southern and eastern parts of the Region are inadequately or poorly served. Services in Mediterranean towns with a large seasonal influx of tourists are periodically interrupted. Furthermore, a lot of water of drinking quality is lost because of leakage from distribution systems in many cities and rural areas. Many rural areas have too few water connections in the home: about 12% of people still need to go to a public fountain, while more than 3% are served by inadequate systems.

The provision of effective sewage disposal facilities is lagging behind. Some 6% of rural and 1% of urban dwellers are reportedly served by inadequate systems. These relatively small reported figures should not serve to hide other problems. Even where people have access to flush toilets, this creates wastewater that must be collected, treated and disposed of or reused. Many towns still lack appropriate sewerage networks, many dwellings in the suburbs are not connected to such systems, and domestic and industrial pollutants are often discharged untreated into the aquatic environment. Concern has been expressed in some instances about the unsafe disposal of the sludge produced by wastewater treatment plants.

Deficiencies in the disposal of wastewater can result in a wide range of organic and inorganic pollutants reaching fertile soils, drinking-water sources and recreational waters. This creates a health risk for the population exposed to contaminated food or water.

Both economic and population growth are increasing the domestic, industrial, agricultural and recreational demand for clean water. The low price of water further encourages its use. At the same time, water is becoming increasingly scarce because of the climatic changes that are taking place in the Region. Unless proper pricing, conservation, surveillance and control measures are instituted, pollution is likely to increase.

International collaboration   Not all countries have comprehensive water policies. When rivers cross or constitute international borders, or where large water sources are shared by countries, international collaboration becomes essential. This is particularly the case in the implementation of international agreements and conventions.

Microbial contamination   Water-related diseases, especially diarrhoeal diseases, are a major cause of death in young children in the poorer countries of the Region. Enteric diseases and hepatitis A have been associated with swimming in polluted lake and sea waters. The consumption of seafood harvested from contaminated areas has also resulted in many cases of infection. Waterborne diseases can thus pose a major threat to tourism and damage exports.

The risk from parasites (particularly *Cryptosporidium*) and viruses in the water supply is widely known. The presence of these pathogens in drinking-water may be responsible for sporadic cases of disease as well as for large outbreaks. Unfortunately, many of these organisms are difficult to detect and are resistant to the disinfectants normally used in the water industry.

Chemical contamination   Lead is often found in older water pipes. There is evidence of its detrimental effects on health, including children's intellectual performance.

Excess concentrations of certain naturally occurring substances, such as arsenic, may pose health problems.

Suggested solutions   The European Charter on Environment and Health *(1)* urges Member States to take all necessary steps to provide adequate water and sanitation.

The International Drinking Water Supply and Sanitation Decade has demonstrated the value of an international approach, in an area where the technical solutions are generally known and where

problems often cross national boundaries. The need for a common Region-wide strategy for the post-Decade period should therefore be considered.

Countries will be able to build on the drinking-water coverage already achieved during the Water Decade, and should give more attention to supplies in rural areas and to the quality of drinking-water. They can define explicit and attainable levels of services appropriate to their specific needs.

Emphasis should also be laid on the appropriate treatment of wastewater and the protection of groundwaters by preventing pollution and leakage of potentially toxic materials.

In many parts of the Region, safe drinking-water has been taken for granted and provided free of charge. The increasing scarcity of water of good quality may require the introduction of charges. These could recover the cost of investments from both users and polluters, as part of water conservation policies to balance the priorities of different water users.

National strategies should aim to provide the whole population with safe drinking-water, by managing and maintaining its collection, treatment and distribution. Effective legislative, administrative and technical measures are also needed for the surveillance and control of pollution of surface water and groundwater and for the protection of fresh and marine waters from pollution. Monitoring and information management should be reinforced to allow rational planning, implementation and evaluation of the actions taken.

Considerable technical knowledge about water already exists. Research could therefore concentrate on developing technologies to investigate the risk factors associated with the presence of pollutants, such as lead or *Cryptosporidium*. Research could also look into lowering the costs of the construction, operation and maintenance of water and wastewater systems.

There is ample scope for international solidarity.

All coastal countries need to reach agreement on the development and implementation of measures to protect the quality of seawater, particularly in areas with bathing beaches or where seafood is harvested. Countries that share water resources also need to develop protocols and agreements on pollution control.

Target 21 – Air quality

By the year 2000, air quality in all countries should be improved to a point at which recognized air pollutants do not pose a threat to public health.

This target can be achieved if all Member States:

- *conduct surveillance of outdoor and indoor air quality;*

- *take appropriate intersectoral action to reduce air pollution originating from industrial and energy production sources, taking account of the WHO air quality guidelines for Europe;*

- *adopt appropriate legislation and administrative and technical measures to control air pollution and comply with criteria for safeguarding human health.*

Problem statement   There are many air pollutants, and they come from various sources. Some pollutants of regional and global significance are sulfur dioxide (SO_2), suspended particulate matter (SPM), nitrogen oxides (NO_x), ozone (O_3), volatile and semivolatile organic compounds (VOC and SVOC) and chlorofluorocarbons (CFC). Some of these, and others such as tobacco smoke, are important for indoor air quality.

SO_2 and SPM   Between 1900 and 1985, global SO_2 emissions from artificial sources increased about sixfold to some 90 million tonnes of sulfur per year, of which about 25% is emitted in the European Region *(5)*. In many countries, local pollution has greatly diminished in recent years. SPM concentration has increased, however, in cities of western and southern Europe. Many urban areas, notably in eastern Europe, have levels of SO_2, SPM and associated

pollutants that are 2 – 4 times the relevant levels of the WHO air quality guidelines for Europe.

NO$_x$ Total emissions of human origin in the Region were estimated to be about 13 million tonnes of nitrogen per year in 1983 *(5)*. Emissions have been increasing in most countries.

Smog episodes Episodically elevated concentrations of air pollution in winter and summer have become common in many cities *(6)*. Two types of smog can be distinguished. The winter-type smog contains SO$_2$ and SPM and stems from the combustion of sulfur-containing fossil fuel. The effects of winter-type smog depend on circumstances and areas. Sulfuric acid is thought to be primarily responsible for the effects on health. The summer-type smog results from photochemical pollution, which arises from atmospheric reactions of hydrocarbons and NO$_x$ stimulated by intense sunlight. In summer-type smog, O$_3$ is considered the biologically most active pollutant.

Global climate change The emission of trace gases and carbon dioxide (CO$_2$) through human activity produces a change in heat radiation from the atmosphere to space, causing the "greenhouse" effect. About 50% of this effect is caused by CO$_2$ and the rest by methane, NO$_x$, O$_3$ in the troposphere and CFC. Some 95% of the global CO$_2$ emissions of human origin arise in the northern hemisphere. Between 1950 and 1984, they increased about three-fold, to an estimated carbon emission of 5300 million tonnes per year. The release of CO$_2$ from deforestation is second only to fossil-fuel combustion as an artificial source. The present global concentration of CO$_2$ is 630 mg/m^3 (350 ppm), which is 25% higher than at the beginning of the industrial revolution, when it was only 500 mg/m^3 (280 ppm).

Ozone layer depletion The O$_3$ layer provides a screen that protects living organisms from the harmful effects of ultraviolet (UV) radiation. When the artificial stable CFC and halons are transported to the stratosphere, they react with and remove O$_3$. The large increase in production of CFC in the early 1970s has now been reduced.

Ozone layer depletion, resulting in increased UV-B radiation at the earth's surface, may seriously damage human health through skin cancer and melanoma, suppression of the immune system and cataracts. Sizeable effects can also be felt by agricultural crops and aquatic ecosystems. A full overview of the possible magnitude of these effects cannot yet be given.

High concentrations of urban air pollutants, such as SO$_2$ and SPM, increase respiratory symptoms, morbidity and mortality. Evidence also suggests that increases in cancer mortality are associated with exposures to polynuclear aromatic hydrocarbons (PAH), benzene and possibly other carcinogens. Heavy metal compounds and SVOC have both direct and indirect (through the food chain and drinking-water) effects on health, depending on the specific pollutant.

The reduction in recent years of local pollution by SO$_2$ and SPM has resulted, in many countries, in a reduction in the incidence of bronchial conditions and an increase in winter sunshine.

Air pollution from road traffic – NO$_x$, particles in diesel fumes and lead – can have adverse effects on health, particularly in urban areas and close to busy main roads.

Indoor air quality   Most people in the Region spend most of their time indoors, but few of the substances commonly found in indoor air have been well studied *(7)*. Since the mid-1970s, the quality of indoor air has been further affected by energy conservation measures, and by changes in building design and in the materials used in construction and in household goods.

The major indoor air pollutant in many places is tobacco smoke. The effects of passive smoking are of special concern. Children of parents who smoke have more respiratory symptoms than children of nonsmoking parents. Evidence shows that regular exposure to environmental tobacco smoke increases the risk of lung cancer and of low birth weight following exposure during gestation *(8)*.

Other major pollutants are radon (associated with an increased risk of lung cancer), viable particles (associated with infectious diseases, including Legionnaires' disease, parasitic diseases and allergic ailments), asbestos and other inorganic fibres (associated with asbestosis, lung cancer and interaction with smoking), formaldehyde (associated with endothelium irritation), and NO_2 and other combustion products, VOC and SVOC (associated with impaired respiratory function and respiratory illness) *(9)*.

Another indoor air quality problem is the "sick building" syndrome. It is associated with the occupancy of large, often newly constructed or remodelled buildings, and is characterized by eye, nose and throat irritation, mental fatigue, headaches, nausea and dizziness. Most of these buildings are workplaces and have forced ventilation systems with partial recirculation of the air and low ventilation rates.

Many cities in the Region are subject to air pollution that directly affects human health. Millions of people are estimated to live in areas where air pollution is severe enough to cause thousands of premature deaths as well as chronic illness and disability each year *(10)*.

If prevention and control measures are not increased, air pollution will get worse. The upward trends in pollution are fuelled by economic growth. Increasing industrialization (producing SO_2, SPM, NO_x, CO_2, heavy metals, SVOC and CFC), more intensive agriculture (producing SPM and NO_x), more vehicle traffic (producing NO_x and SO_2) and more domestic heating (producing CO_2) all contribute. Rapidly increasing urbanization means even faster deterioration of environmental conditions in cities.

Fortunately, the signs are that pollution trends can be reversed. Industrial emissions have been considerably reduced, particularly in northern and western Europe, thanks to more effective controls and the closure of many older factories. In some heavily industrialized areas, however, especially in eastern Europe where soft brown coal is used in a high proportion of domestic heating and power generation, pollution levels remain high.

The production and release of CFC peaked in 1974. The subsequent decline is due to consumer education and restrictions on non-essential uses in several countries.

Several countries have introduced incentives or regulations to reduce the exhaust emissions of cars, but increased traffic density has often counterbalanced this reduction.

Suggested solutions   The European Charter on Environment and Health *(1)* urges Member

States to pay attention to air quality and to observe the WHO air quality guidelines for Europe *(4)*. Of particular concern are the oxides of sulfur and nitrogen, the photochemical oxidants (summer-type smog) and VOC, as well as radon and tobacco smoke in indoor air.

An air quality policy should address the many agencies responsible for action. Its aim is to strengthen the legislative, economic and technical measures that should reduce national and local air pollution at least to the levels of the WHO air quality guidelines for Europe. The control of long-range transboundary air pollutants, such as SO_2 and NO_x, needs effective international agreements. Given the generally unfavourable trends in pollution, action should not await additional studies. Measures to reduce emissions from industry, domestic premises and motor vehicles and substantially to reduce indoor air pollutants should be introduced immediately.

In cities, the simultaneous and well managed reduction and control of all the major sources of air pollution (energy production, manufacturing industry, incinerators, vehicles and the indoor environment) would greatly enhance the health image and attractiveness of the city – both to its own citizens and to visitors. The improvements produced by cleaner air were demonstrated conclusively in the London area in the 1960s, thanks to the introduction of legislation.

A number of Member States have already taken specific action that will reduce environmental and health risks. Such action should, therefore, be expanded and includes, among others, the development and use of low-polluting alternative energy sources, the use of alternative raw materials or technologies or the modification of production processes, a faster reduction of and more extensive restrictions on the production and use of CFC and halons, and continued intensified action on air pollution from vehicles.

Indoor air quality would be improved by the promotion of smoke-free schools, worksites and public places. More attention to construction design and building materials would reduce the hazard from radon, various organic compounds and biological contaminants. The improvement of ventilation in general, and the elimination of unvented heaters and cooking stoves, reduces the products of combustion indoors.

The WHO air quality guidelines for Europe need to be revised and expanded periodically, as new evidence becomes available. This will make them of consistent use in countries and internationally, as a benchmark for the development of comprehensive and effective air quality control laws and regulations.

A better knowledge and information base is also needed. Perhaps least is known about many of the indoor air pollutants. In the case of other pollutants, studies are needed to improve the understanding of the short- and long-term interrelation between air quality and human health, so as to develop and improve action strategies in cities and elsewhere.

Research might look at: the measurement and assessment of personal and population exposures and quantitative exposure – response relationships; models of air pollution emission and dispersion throughout the Region and assessments of population exposure; and, in selected areas, quantitative risk assessment on the basis of actual human exposures and exposure – response relationships.

Target 22 – Food quality and safety

By the year 2000, health risks due to microorganisms or their toxins, to chemicals and to radioactivity in food should have been significantly reduced in all Member States.

This target can be achieved if the appropriate bodies in all Member States:

- *introduce effective legislative, administrative and technical measures for the surveillance and control of food contamination at all stages of farming, slaughtering, harvesting, food processing, distribution, storage, sale and use;*

- *reduce the mean weekly intake of chemical contaminants to or below the WHO guideline values for permissible weekly intakes;*

- *inform consumers on the composition of food;*

- *achieve full reporting of outbreaks of foodborne intestinal diseases;*

- *promote awareness of food hygiene and proper nutrition in all persons involved in producing, handling and selling food.*

Problem statement   Methods of food production, storage, distribution and preparation are rapidly changing. The international trade in food and tourism is expected to expand rapidly, owing both to the political opening of the central and eastern part of the Region and to the establishment of a single market without trade barriers in the European Community countries. Changing social habits and the entry of a large proportion of women into the labour market all over Europe have led to changes in the pattern of food consumption, as mass catering increasingly replaces home cooking. These changes bring with them new problems of food hygiene and transboundary infections and intoxications. In addition to being a potential health hazard, unsafe food may have serious economic consequences for food exports and tourism.

Chemical contamination   The current levels of common chemical contaminants in individual foods and in total diet in most countries of the Region are generally well within the established WHO guidelines for exposure limits. With the exception of most of the countries in the central and eastern part of the Region, the trend is generally downward, as the use of persistent pesticides and environmental pollution with other toxic chemicals is curtailed or banned altogether. Food additives used to improve the quality and appearance of foods undergo systematic toxicological evaluation.

In some situations, however, specific population groups may be unduly exposed. Considerable contamination of food still occurs, including organochlorine pesticides and PCBs in human milk, mercury and PCBs in fish, lead in canned foods and aflatoxins in nuts and cereals.

A number of dramatic incidents involving the chemical or radioactive contamination of foods have created considerable concern in the Region. A well known example is the toxic oil syndrome in Spain, which killed some people and seriously impaired the health of many others. Another well known incident is the Chernobyl nuclear accident in the USSR.

Microbiological contamination Foodborne diseases have increased over the last few years and have reached epidemic proportions in several countries. The main infections are with *Salmonella* (especially *S. enteritidis*) and *Campylobacter* strains. The current reported incidence rate of over 1200 cases per million inhabitants in the Region is about three times higher than that recorded in 1984. Since only a few of the acute cases of gastrointestinal infections are reported in most countries, the number of cases should probably be multiplied by at least 10. Diarrhoeal diseases and other foodborne infections and intoxications are still the most important and frequent form of illness in tourists.

Food safety services The structure, staffing and organization of national food safety services vary widely across the Region, reflecting the different social, political and economic circumstances under which they were developed. In most countries, two or more central government departments share responsibility without appropriate intersectoral collaboration. This leaves some areas with ill-defined preventive strategies and inappropriately implemented control measures. In addition, few countries have a comprehensive food policy that includes health, the environment and the economy.

For the last 30 years, the Joint FAO/WHO Expert Committee on Food Additives and the Joint FAO/WHO Meeting on Pesticide Residues have played a major role in making safety assessments of different chemicals in food. These two committees develop exposure limits for chemicals in food, under the mandate of the Codex Alimentarius programme *(11)*. Their recommendations are based on the WHO principles and criteria for the safety evaluation of food additives and contaminants *(12)* and pesticide residues *(13)*. Significant progress has been made in legislative measures, based on this work.

By contrast, important gaps remain in information and communication. Communication with the trade and the general public about unsafe food and drinks is not always effective, within countries or internationally. The difficulty of clear and informative communication was demonstrated by the Chernobyl nuclear accident. Initial uncertainties about the nature and extent of the accident and inadequate intersectoral contingency planning resulted in confused messages to the public. The measures imposed in Europe to safeguard foodstuffs were often contradictory. Valid information about the dietary intakes of population groups was not available, making it difficult to assess the real impact on health of contaminated food.

Suggested solutions A new approach to food safety has to be found if the vicious circle of food contamination and foodborne disease is to be broken. More legislation, more standards and more inspection and food control alone are not the answer. Rather, the appropriate strategy would sustain food safety as part of a comprehensive food quality policy. It would strengthen international, national and local programmes for the monitoring of food contamination and the surveillance of foodborne diseases. It would also harmonize the education and training of food safety personnel, and implement policies of intersectoral collaboration in food safety.

As people become better informed, they can be expected to demand food of higher quality that is both safe and nutritious. Meeting this demand will require a closer link between the professional, scientific and commercial networks in the hitherto quite separate fields of food safety and nutrition.

A special effort needs to be made to help the countries in the central and eastern part of the Region to cope with food safety problems.

Information and monitoring   Food safety requires stronger epidemiological services, accurate, adequate and comparable information, and better countrywide programmes for the monitoring and surveillance of food contamination and foodborne diseases.

Emphasis should be given to the epidemiological investigation of outbreaks of foodborne diseases, laboratory investigations and early warning systems so as to harmonize European efforts in food safety, as part of the WHO Surveillance Programme for Control of Foodborne Infections and Intoxications in Europe. These efforts should include population investigations and sentinel studies on infectious intestinal diseases, so as to assess the real incidence and assist risk management.

Monitoring requires agreed standards of sampling, methods of analysis and analytical quality, and a consistent submission of data on agreed contaminants and foods. Further, scientifically valid dietary intake studies are needed to interpret data and assess people's exposure to hazardous chemicals and the associated potential risk. Such studies could be adapted for the European Region from studies carried out elsewhere by the Food and Agriculture Organization of the United Nations (FAO), WHO and UNEP. The 1990 European Conference on Food and Nutrition Policy *(14)* requested FAO, WHO and other international and national agencies to study the feasibility and cost of creating reliable and accessible European sources of information on food and nutrition.

The safety aspects of food could be adequately and cost-effectively controlled by further developing and applying a programme that relies on the control of selected critical points through hazard analysis rather than end-product testing. Specific training programmes could usefully be developed for food inspectors, food technologists and caterers. Human resource development in general would benefit from permanent European training programmes for trainers.

Food hygiene and safety require communication with the general public and the food business that is both clear and informative. Only then can unnecessary food scares be avoided and people, industry and trade be mobilized to undertake prompt and effective prevention and control.

The World Health Assembly, in resolution WHA42.40, called for an intensification of international action to prevent and control foodborne diseases. In the European Region, this includes intensifying collaboration between the various intergovernmental organizations already active in food safety and related aspects of food quality.

Target 23 – Waste management and soil pollution

By the year 2000, public health risks caused by solid and hazardous wastes and soil pollution should be effectively controlled in all Member States.

This target can be achieved if all Member States:

- *introduce effective legislative, administrative and technical measures for the management of solid municipal and hazardous wastes;*

- *introduce effective measures for soil conservation and the rehabilitation of polluted soil;*

- *adopt effective measures to eliminate the health risks due to accumulation of waste and soil pollution.*

Problem statement Owing to its physical, chemical or biological characteristics, hazardous waste requires special handling and disposal procedures to avoid risk to health or adverse environmental effects.

Most hazardous waste originates from the manufacturing industry and the use of chemicals. Medical waste, such as that from hospitals, and certain wastes from research laboratories are also hazardous. Radioactive waste is clearly a major health hazard.

Municipal waste More municipal waste is generated each year *(15)*. In London, it increased between 1968 and 1982 by some 25%, to about 0.4 tonnes per person per year *(8)*. In the Netherlands in 1986, the figure was about 1 tonne per person per year *(5)*. In the whole European Region, several hundred million tonnes of waste are generated each

year. To this figure must be added industrial and construction waste, surplus manure, polluted soil and, for some countries, dredging sludge. Together, the total waste that needs handling and disposal may amount to several thousand million tonnes per year. Municipal waste disposal is likely be one of the most significant problems for many cities in the 1990s and hence a major issue for the health of cities.

Many countries have taken action to control the disposal of waste, including domestic legislation in line with important directives from the European Community. Nevertheless, problems remain. A number of major incidents in recent years have resulted in gross contamination of soil and groundwater. In many less dramatic cases, unsatisfactory methods have led to a gradual build-up of pollution as well as to occasional health hazards. Clandestine disposal in rivers and public sewers sometimes occurs, often involving hazardous waste.

In some countries, pesticides are often handled without proper care and partly filled containers may be left to rot. Facilities are not always available for the collection and safe disposal of hazardous consumer products such as waste oil and household chemicals. Potentially toxic materials are still occasionally transported and stored without clear labelling and without adequate precautions to prevent spills or seepage. Some countries have no arrangements for educating users about potential dangers.

Soil pollution   Soil pollution is a growing concern for countries of the Region. The increasing pollution of urban and agricultural soils by toxic chemicals with a high absorption capacity, such as heavy metals and dioxins, has direct consequences for human health, food safety and groundwater quality. The sources of soil pollution are spills, the deposition of air pollutants, the excessive spread of chemicals used in agriculture, and the improper disposal of liquid and solid wastes on land. Agricultural soil pollution may reduce yields while increasing the concentration of unwanted chemicals in crops for human consumption and animal feed. The infiltration of the chemicals into groundwater aquifers endangers water resources and complicates their preparation for drinking-water supply.

The problem of soil pollution is exacerbated by high stack dispersion of air pollutants over large areas, the sludge and slurries applied to land, and the disposal of waste in landfills. In some areas, pollutants have accumulated in soil to such a level that it is losing its agricultural fertility.

Some central, eastern and southern European countries (such as Bulgaria, the Czech Republic, Greece,

Poland, Romania and Slovakia) have identified soil pollution as a serious environmental health problem. In some western European areas, such as Brittany in France, the soil is reaching saturation point for the disposal of pig manure. In other places, the disposal of sludge and slurries on land has irreversibly reduced the quality of water aquifers.

If present trends continue, more food of unsafe quality will be grown and more land may be completely lost to agriculture. Intoxication of children, especially lead poisoning caused by dust from polluted urban soil, will increase and the quality of rural drinking-water will continue to deteriorate. These are all symptoms of a failure to recognize that soils have a limited capacity to absorb and deal with contaminants.

Waste disposal   The uncontrolled handling and disposal of hazardous waste may be a danger to health. Waste collection, transport and handling may be an occupational health hazard for workers. Disposal, dumping, storage or incineration may, if carried out improperly or ineffectively, cause hazards to health by polluting the environment. The transfrontier transport of hazardous waste increases these risks and adds the problem of less competent handling of the waste far from its source.

Waste reduction   Waste is inevitably produced by industrial processes and by municipalities. Public concern initially focused on particular types of hazardous waste, such as those produced by industry and hospitals. More recently, the public desire for a less wasteful society has begun to turn industrial production towards low-waste technologies. Although the incentives of resource recovery and energy conservation are leading to greater recycling and reuse, the quantities of waste that require disposal are still expanding in most countries.

Information   The quality and availability of waste disposal statistics are extremely variable. Information about the total quantities of municipal waste countries dispose of, the type and amount of waste disposed of per person and changes in the importance of the two major disposal options, landfill and incineration, is very limited and available only to some countries in the Region. Industrial and hazardous waste disposal cannot yet be well quantified because of variations in the definitions of the waste and different methods of reporting the data. In spite of the knowledge accumulated about soil contamination, the impact of soil pollution on the health of the public is still not well defined.

Suggested solutions   A waste control policy should cover legislative, administrative, technical and educational measures. These measures should address safe collection, transport, handling, treatment and disposal of both municipal and hazardous wastes, the protection of soil from pollution, and effective international agreements on the transfrontier shipment of hazardous waste.

At the local level, a healthy city policy will include waste prevention, control and disposal. It is good practice to inform the population about the size of the problem and the options for its solution, to educate the public on new technological and managerial developments, and to encourage every individual and business establishment to support sound municipal waste management. Rural areas also need policies on waste and soil pollution.

While landfill remains an important method of waste disposal, the selection of sites is becoming more difficult. Therefore, greater use of incineration and energy recovery is necessary as an alternative form of waste management. Waste prevention and reuse must also be encouraged, to further reduce the need for space.

Prevention means that waste is not created. Non-waste or low-waste solutions and technologies should be developed and used. Today, the decision to prevent waste is often made on the basis of economic considerations alone. A health objective, such as preventing the release of certain environmentally harmful substances, can be more effective. When another process or another raw material produces less hazardous waste, and the cost of the change is covered by savings in the cost of removal, prevention becomes economically attractive.

Reuse is the useful application of waste products in the same or another process. Technical measures include the recycling of waste, the manufacture of useful by-products, alternative methods of production or the selection of alternative raw materials. In principle, this provides secondary raw materials to replace primary raw materials. The chances are that these secondary products will cost appreciably less than primary raw materials, although sometimes this is because reuse is subsidized. Their quality and properties, of course, also play a role.

In the next decade or two, the reuse of municipal waste could be increased by about 50% if the organic fraction was collected separately and more paper, cardboard, glass, metal, plastics and textiles were recycled. To be fully effective, such separation should start at each individual source.

Some 50% more reuse of course waste also appears possible because almost 70% of the total consists of paper, bulky waste, cardboard, metal and wood. The reuse of construction and demolition waste can be increased to 80% by better separation of its components at the building site. Only little improvement is possible with industrial waste, because levels of recycling are already high. It may be possible to recycle up to 25% of office, shop and service sector waste. About 20% of all waste must be incinerated, including old tyres. This has the benefit of producing energy but care must be taken not to increase air pollution by inappropriate or ineffective means of incineration. With maximal reuse and recycling, only 15% of waste will have to be disposed of in landfills, requiring an area that is some 40% less than at present (16).

Hence, the primary indicator and standard for the magnitude of the removal problem could be seen as the space required for waste that cannot be processed further. In addition, for some priority substances, the level of emissions from waste incinerators should be the key measure. This applies in particular to persistent substances such as metals, PCBs, dioxins and furans.

Other measures that some countries have found useful involve encouraging manufacturers and packers to reduce the quantities of household waste (40% by weight is waste packaging) and industrial waste, to design waste materials that are readily recoverable and recyclable, and to avoid non-treatable composite materials. Another measure has been to integrate into town plans the sites and systems required to introduce selective collection.

Measures can be taken to reduce emissions and should be used to a greater extent at disposal and incineration plants. Air pollution control at the source, the optimum use of chemicals in agriculture and the safe disposal of waste will decrease soil pollution. Some polluted soils may be rehabilitated by incineration and destruction of the toxic chemicals they contain. Of course, the agricultural fertility of such soils would have to be regenerated. The handling and rehabilitation of abandoned polluted land in former industrial areas around big cities will require special attention.

Better information is needed about soil pollution and the public health problems associated with it. The main sources of pollution require investigation, whether they are the deposition of air pollutants, the indiscriminate spreading of chemicals, landfilling or waste applied to land.

The handling of hazardous waste should follow internationally agreed procedures, including limiting transfrontier transport to the minimum, while following the principle that hazardous waste should be taken care of by its generator, as close to its generation point as possible. In principle, all countries should aim to be self-sufficient in waste disposal capability.

Target 24 – Human ecology and settlements

By the year 2000, cities, towns and rural communities throughout the Region should offer physical and social environments supportive to the health of their inhabitants.

This target can be achieved if intersectoral, ecological approaches combining community planning and public health are used to improve the built environment and if countries take action to:

- *ensure active community participation in determining needs and problems, and in the processes of planning and action;*

- *adopt community planning approaches that emphasize ecological concerns and the needs of people and facilitate social interaction in all human settlements;*

- *strengthen programmes for the construction of healthy houses and housing improvement, including proper sanitation facilities and the provision of open spaces and recreational areas;*

- *meet the needs of special groups such as young families, the old and people with disabilities;*

- *introduce measures for intersectoral action to mobilize the support and resources of all sectors in community improvement;*

- *reach agreement on international health criteria for community planning and development, including housing, management of domestic waste, noise control and safety, and strengthen legislative, administrative and technical measures and services.*

Problem statement Most people in the Region now live in towns. Structural changes in commerce and industry have resulted in more inner-city unemployment, poverty, and decay. Housing tends to be a particular problem for certain groups of the population. For example, housing is often poor for elderly people, specially those who are physically frail, in poor health, living alone or in need of some supervision *(17)*.

The percentage of homeless or unsuitably housed people is reported by only a few countries and varies considerably, largely because of diverse national definitions of standard accommodation.

The central and eastern part of the Region, in particular, not only has heavily polluted cities but also has rural communities with hazardous environmental conditions, poor water supply and sanitation facilities, intensive pollution by agricultural chemicals, soil pollution from air pollutants or the land disposal of wastes, and problems linked to manure disposal especially from giant pig feedlots.

Social and living environments tend to go hand in hand and have a combined impact on health and wellbeing. If present trends continue, inequities will increase, especially inequalities in access to a healthy living environment.

Many people in the Region spend less than 20% of their time in the open air and thus the indoor environment has a particularly important effect on health. New methods of construction and new materials for furniture and fittings, together with more effective thermal insulation, have raised the levels of potentially harmful contaminants indoors. Radon in houses is a major problem in some areas of the Region and is probably second only to smoking as a contributor to the incidence of lung cancer. Conversely, many of the poorer sections of the population live in badly insulated houses with inadequate heating. Elderly people living alone are particularly prone to hypothermia.

Waste collection from houses is now general throughout most of the Region, particularly in urban areas. Difficulties in the final disposal of waste have increased in recent years, however, because of a growing shortage of suitable land, and problems of scavenging, composting and incineration.

Community noise has greatly increased in many areas. Unwanted noise causes stress and may cause physical impairment at high decibel levels.

Community involvement in promoting environmental health in housing is rarely reported, and its role appears limited.

Suggested solutions   As the WHO Healthy Cities movement has shown, a holistic policy is needed to improve health and socioeconomic development in urban and rural communities. The strategy will differ from country to country.

In western Europe, attention should be paid to reestablishing a social environment supportive to health, especially in deprived areas and underprivileged suburbs of big cities.

In many areas in southern Europe, the first priority remains to rehabilitate substandard housing and improve the physical environment in the urban fringes of quickly growing cities.

In the central and eastern part of the Region, one priority will be to reduce gross pollution levels, especially air and soil pollution in major industrial cities. Another will be to improve environmental conditions in rural areas by upgrading the water supply, sanitation facilities and housing standards, by better control of the use of agricultural chemicals, by better management of animal waste, and by the rehabilitation of derelict land. This will also help to rehabilitate agricultural production and improve nutrition and food safety.

Every country requires political will at both national and local government levels to reverse unhealthy living conditions and inequities in access to a healthy living environment. Local governments know their particular circumstances. They should therefore be encouraged to mobilize their own and their community's resources to improve health, social and environmental conditions. Experience in Oslo and other cities has shown the usefulness of all residents participating in making their neighbourhoods healthy.

Several western European countries are attempting to provide a more supportive and healthy socioeconomic environment by directing urbanization away from the larger conurbations. Some countries (notably France, Germany, the Netherlands and the United Kingdom) have paid special attention to ethnic minority groups with low incomes, who may constitute a sizeable proportion or even a majority of the population in certain areas. They require urban development policies that are sensitive to their needs, particularly in terms of affordable and decent housing. In the central and eastern part of the Region, countries have long-term strategies that aim both at improving housing standards and at modernizing the existing housing stock.

Pedestrian and cycle paths, parks and playgrounds are important incentives for regular physical activity and social interaction. These amenities, as well as efficient rubbish collection and the absence of traffic fumes and noise, all contribute to health and wellbeing and should be more widely available. The brutal urban architecture of the 1960s is being replaced by styles that appear to create a greater sense of wellbeing and belonging. Accident prevention in both homes and streets remains an important element of health promotion in the urban environment.

Methods of dealing with community noise include trying to increase public awareness of the harmful effects of noise, and reducing noise by means of building and traffic regulations and town planning.

Developments in housing include legislation (on asbestos, formaldehyde and radon, for example), the establishment of housing criteria, and greater emphasis on the housing of vulnerable groups, particularly elderly and disabled people, including sheltered housing. International health criteria for community planning and development also need to be strengthened.

Housing can be an important support to social networks and to the integration of three or more generations of families. In Denmark and in several other countries, regulations on new housing call for easy access for the physically handicapped, and for the provision of areas for leisure activities. In Sweden it is estimated that, of the more than 100 000 elderly people living in institutions, over half could live on their own with suitable support. A law on housing aims to reduce the number of institutional beds by 50 000 by the year 2000.

The Falköping accident prevention programme in Sweden, developed on the basis of intervention and evaluation in the community, has brought about a 25 – 30% decrease in local accidents *(18)*.

Research Three research topics will be of vital importance in the long run. One is the study of the health impact of trends in the economic and social development of our societies, particularly in energy production, agriculture, industry, transport and urbanization. Another is the study of the effects of the environment on health, which can inform urban development plans and architectural projects. The third is interdisciplinary research into human ecology, involving public health and environmental health institutes and the human ecology departments of universities. In addition, a number of scientific studies may improve knowledge in specific subjects, such as indoor air pollution, allergens in the indoor environment, the sick building syndrome, the mental health aspects of housing and local environments, the interaction of family and other supportive environments, and ways of involving the public.

Target 25 – Health of people at work

By the year 2000, the health of workers in all Member States should be improved by making work environments more healthy, reducing work-related disease and injury, and promoting the wellbeing of people at work.

This target can be achieved if effective measures are implemented in all Member States that:

- *reduce disease, injury, disability and absence from work resulting from exposures to workplace hazards such as dust, noise, chemicals and stress;*

- *ensure that all employees have access to occupational health services;*

- *facilitate the adoption of work practices and routines that contribute to the health and wellbeing of workers;*

- *promote healthy lifestyles such as healthy nutrition, physical exercise and non-smoking;*

- *promote cooperation between relevant interest groups and sectors such as labour, industry, environment, education and health, and with the International Labour Office and other relevant international bodies, in the formulation and implementation of strategies.*

Problem statement   In the European Region, health policies directed at the workplace are still mainly confined to the prevention of occupational disease and injury, with minor medical care for workers in some places. Attempts to integrate occupational health with primary health care and health promotion are rare, owing to separate organizational structures, lack of appropriate mechanisms for procedure or insufficient occupational health expertise among primary health care workers.

Occupational health services   People at work are not comprehensively covered by occupational health activities. Of about 100 000 physicians in occupational health in the European Region, about one third to one half are full time. Of about 172 500 occupational health nurses, about 60 000 have been specifically trained in occupational health and two thirds work on a full-time basis. Over 100 million workers in transport, agriculture, small industries and construction, or in remote areas, remain without easy access to occupational health services. Many others, such as the self-employed, are not covered by services at all. Only about 45% of the economically active population in the Region as a whole are estimated to be covered by in-plant or group occupational health services, while a further 30% are covered by more limited occupational health services linked to primary health care. Coverage varies greatly between countries, ranging from less than 10% to almost 100% of the economically active population *(19)*.

Occupational disease and accidents   Prevention has focused on the early detection of occupational disease, and the exposure to many toxic agents and harmful physical factors at work has been reduced. Nevertheless, workers in the Region are exposed to a wide range of occupational health and safety hazards, with an estimated 10.6 million accidents at work yearly, 21 000 of which are fatal. Many of these are preventable. Some 650 000 new cases of occupational disease are estimated to occur annually within the European Region, with an average annual incidence of 1.85 per 1000 workers *(19)*. In the future, as living and working environments increasingly blend, the rates of some occupational diseases will gradually adjust to the levels found in the general population of working age.

Economic implications   The cost of work days lost due to work injury such as trauma, low-back problems and musculoskeletal damage runs into billions of dollars and continues to grow. Their cost to health care budgets is staggering (US $20 thousand million per year in the United States) and remains without question a priority issue. Lost days due to employee illness reach high figures. In the Region, hundreds of millions of work days are lost annually, causing unnecessary human suffering and costing nations thousands of millions of dollars a year.

Large numbers of the Region's total workforce – almost half the population – are also burdened by chronic disorders such as diabetes, visual and hearing impairments, cardiovascular diseases, infectious diseases, genetic disorders, cancers and sexually transmitted diseases. In addition, many of the environmental hazards to which the general population is exposed – such as noise, chemicals and dusts – are 10 to 100 times more concentrated at workplaces. Improvement in the work environment would thus help to reduce external environmental exposure.

Of the present total of 355 million workers active in the European Region, 232 million live and work in the central and eastern part of the Region *(19)*. Employment by sector – services (50%), industry (35%) and agriculture (15%) in the Region as a whole – differs between west and east. A predominance is building up throughout the Region in the service sector. This brings with it the problems of new skills and training, understaffing in other sectors and, in consequence, the risk of more injuries and stress (see also target 1 on aspects of unemployment).

Women   Women's health issues have physiological, biological, sociological, cultural and economic aspects. Probably around 150 million of the 355 million workers in the Region are women, and their share is gradually increasing. This highlights the need, when planning work environments, to consider carefully the differences between the sexes in anthropometry, reproductive functions, physiology and physical activity. The potential effects, such as injury to genetic material, fetotoxicity and the possibly elevated risk of psychomotor morbidity, are problems that justify attention (see also target 8).

Mental health   A number of workplace conditions may cause or trigger psychiatric disorders. The role of stress is well understood. Mental disturbances can also result from exposure to pathogenic substances employed in industrial processes, yet the widespread tendency is still to attribute all such complaints to nerves or hysteria and to neglect the real causes. Low levels of exposure to toxic substances are the rule rather than the exception in modern plants, and careful attention is given to new chemicals released on the market. Nevertheless, long-term exposure is not well studied and experience shows that safety regulations are not always observed. Indeed, situations continue to arise in which workers suffer exposure to toxins, sometimes of a high level *(19)*.

Diet   It is increasingly recognized that dietary modifications can significantly reduce the risk of several major chronic diseases. They can also be a major determinant of the health status and quality of life of a population. Unbalanced nutrient intake and overconsumption (leading to obesity and cardiovascular disease) are issues on which health promotion programmes at workplaces need strengthening, particularly through awareness, information and guidelines.

Communicable disease   Tremendous progress has been made in public health immunization, and sanitation policies have improved the coverage, health and productivity of people at work. Nevertheless, a good proportion of existing occupational morbidity and mortality from such diseases as tetanus and hepatitis B is both costly and preventable.

First aid is a fundamental need in the workplace. It saves lives, limits impairment and reduces disability time and health costs, yet millions of people at work have no access to good first aid.

High-risk occupational groups, who are likely to experience adverse effects earlier than the general population, are not always systematically tracked. Surveillance programmes are not mandatory by law in all countries and wide variation exists in their application and goals.

Vulnerable groups   Age is a developing process and should be valued. Increasing life expectancy means that more elderly people will continue their working life. Their physiological and psychological needs require special attention.

Thousands of children are born disabled or with potential disability each year. As adults they need to be better integrated into the workplace and society, and employers need to increase their recruitment of disabled people. Public health and occupational health services need to make a substantial contribution for people already exercising a skill or profession who become disabled, as a result of work injury or illness. More accurate assessments of disability and clear criteria for early return to work are also needed (see also target 3).

One third of the countries in the Region have achieved advanced levels in workplace conditions. They offer a relatively healthy environment, reduced risk, injury and disease, and good access to occupational health care. Even these are only in the early stages of health promotion, however. Larger industries have increased their investment in workplace health and now provide occupational activities that complement each other in ways that benefit health. In other countries, occupational health services need urgent development to meet expectations, directives, legislation and people's concern for a safe and healthy working environment.

While countries continue to accumulate data on injury and ill health, occupational health information is often irregular, scattered, lacking or not comparable. Difficulties occur with definitions and with sector boundaries, which include health, labour, environment, hygiene and other institutions. The lack of overall coordination, precision and dissemination of data hampers decision-making. In consequence, indicators of the health status of the workplace are as yet poorly developed, and few countries have established a national baseline for workers' health.

Suggested solutions   Many occupations enhance people's physical, mental and social wellbeing. At the same time, work can play an important role in mortality, disease, injury, impairment, disability and psychological strain.

A policy for healthy workplaces should therefore emphasize the importance of preventive strategies that aim to reduce work-related health risks. It should also support healthy practices, including a stimulating job, flexible working hours, health-promoting arrangements, moderate exercise, balanced nutrition, the ability to cope with stress, a lack of sexual and racial harassment, nonsmoking, a moderate use of alcohol and a lack of substance abuse. It could also spell out some economic benefits, such as the reduction in total health care expenditure and the increase in economic competitiveness.

Changes in workplace settings can be made to encourage the adoption of healthy lifestyles. The health and wellbeing of people at work would be enhanced if these issues received early attention.

The principles and concepts being developed for health promotion at work deserve the support of public health authorities, trade unions and employees alike. In Finland and Sweden, pilot studies on occupational health services for small workplaces have recently been carried out and ways of cooperating with primary health care units investigated. Considerable experience of services in small workplaces also exists in France. Practical, large-scale activities to provide services for small undertakings and the self-employed are taking place in Italy.

The economic benefits to firms have already been demonstrated in the United States, where wellbeing programmes have existed for at least 20 years and address exercise, smoking, diet, alcohol and stress. A healthy company is typically also a wealthy company. In view of the long lead time for chronic diseases, the full impact of today's positive health promotion at the workplace will be seen beyond the year 2000. Health promotion in the workplace needs to be backed up by high-quality studies and reviews, as well as educational programmes for the professions emerging in this field.

One aim of occupational health services is to cover all workplaces effectively. The organization and functions of occupational health services in the Region vary in many respects. In every case, comprehensive services require adequate support systems. These may be structured in different ways, depending on local circumstances. They are likely to include the surveillance of physical and mental illness caused or aggravated by work injury, work processes and exposure; health promotion; reporting and data collection; advisory services for employers and employees; effective management; and collaboration between labour and management. Specially important is the development of a methodology and public policies for the organization of health services for small industries and for the self-employed, with easy access for those with special needs. The overall needs of women in the workplace need to be more clearly identified and policies for their implementation urgently established.

Irrespective of the existing systems of funding for occupational health services, formal support and incentives would increase the coverage and improve the service. Discussions should take place to develop the methodology and administrative process required for interaction between occupational health care and primary health care. The services should add up to a national network that would link institutions, industry, relevant government sectors and national experts. They should facilitate the concerted input of data on workers' health, as well as research, comparability and effective decision-making. They should also identify new needs and generate new measures to deal with them, disseminate knowledge, and increase the exchange of expertise within and outside the national boundaries.

More and better educated occupational health staff of all disciplines are needed to offer training, education, decision-making, implementation, diagnosis and support services to meet the emerging needs in the years ahead.

The health of workers depends heavily on team activities involving a number of different professionals. They therefore need a high level of knowledge of their own discipline and a core knowledge of that of other members of the team. All the members need a wider understanding of public health and environmental policies, as well as good management practice at all stages and levels. Educational curricula and teaching methods should be developed to meet the evolving requirements of these team professionals in the years to come.

Better national occupational health databases are needed. Baselines can then be identified from which targets for an appropriate and feasible reduction of existing major illness and injury can be developed. Measurements should be comparable throughout the Region, and consequently lead to the development of a valuable regional database for trends in Europe.

Changing personal behaviour is a sensitive matter. Effective outcomes can only result from an informed workforce with a right to know and with health support and participation at all levels. Participation, health risks, attitudes and behaviour need to be reflected better in the education and awareness of workers. The formulation and implementation of strategies require proper legal foundations, as well as cooperation with interest groups, with other sectors of government and the economy, and with the International Labour Office, the European Community and other relevant international bodies.

References

1. *Environment and health. The European Charter and commentary.* Copenhagen, WHO Regional Office for Europe, 1990 (WHO Regional Publications, European Series, No. 35).
2. *Sundsvall statement on supportive environments for health. Third International Conference on Health Promotion.* Geneva, World Health Organization, 1992 (document WHO/HED/92.1).
3. *Guidelines for drinking-water quality* (Vol. 1, 2 & 3). Geneva, World Health Organization, 1984 & 1985.
4. *Air quality guidelines for Europe.* Copenhagen, WHO Regional Office for Europe, 1987 (WHO Regional Publications, European Series, No. 23).

5. United Nations Environment Programme, *Environmental data report*. Oxford, Basil Blackwell, 1987.

6. *Acute effects on health of smog episodes*. Report on a WHO meeting. Copenhagen, WHO Regional Office for Europe, 1992 (WHO Regional Publications, European Series, No. 43).

7. *Health aspects related to indoor air quality: report on a WHO Working Group*. Copenhagen, WHO Regional Office for Europe, 1979 (EURO Reports and Studies, No. 21).

8. VAN OYEN, H.J. *Health for all in Europe: an epidemiological review*. Copenhagen, WHO Regional Office for Europe, 1990 (document EUR/ICP/HSC 013(6)/BD/1).

9. *Working group on indoor air quality: inorganic fibres and other particulate matter*. Copenhagen, WHO Regional Office for Europe, 1991 (document EUR/ICP/CEH 096(S)).

10. *Impact on human health of air pollution in Europe*. Copenhagen, WHO Regional Office for Europe, 1991 (document EUR/ICP/CEH 097).

11. *Codex Alimentarius*. Abridged version. Rome, Food and Agriculture Organization, 1990.

12. *Principles for the safety assessment of food additives and contaminants in food*. Geneva, World Health Organization, 1987 (Environmental Health Criteria, No. 70).

13. *Principles for the toxicological assessment of pesticide residues in food*. Geneva, World Health Organization, 1990 (Environmental Health Criteria, No. 104).

14. *Food and nutrition policy in Europe*: report on a WHO Conference. Copenhagen, WHO Regional Office for Europe, 1991 (document EUR/ICP/NUT 133).

15. PESCOD, M.B., ED. *Urban solid waste management*. Florence, IRIS, 1991.

16. LANGEWED, F., ED. *Concern for tomorrow. A national environmental survey 1985 – 2010*. Bilthoven, National Institute of Public Health and Environmental Protection, 1989.

17. RANSON, R. *Healthy housing: a practical guide*. London, E. & F.N. Spon, 1991.

18. SCHELP, L. *Community intervention and accidents. Epidemiology as a basis for evaluation of a community intervention programme on accidents*. Stockholm, Karolinska Institute, 1987.

19. RANTANEN, J., ED. *Occupational health services: an overview*. Copenhagen, WHO Regional Office for Europe, 1990 (WHO Regional Publications, European Series, No. 26).

6

Appropriate care

Health services are attracting increasingly close attention and budgetary scrutiny in most Member States. Chapters 4 and 5 focused on policies, programmes and specific activities that can contribute significantly to the improvement of health and the prevention of disease by promoting and supporting healthy patterns of living and by ameliorating the environment. These initiatives are complemented by developments in the provision of comprehensive health services of good quality that are accessible to the whole population. This is the third essential area of action in the regional health for all policy, and this chapter deals with the main issues involved. Health care functions include not only curative care but also:

- the maintenance and development of prevention services in such fields as immunization and the surveillance of child growth and development;
- the provision of screening, early detection and treatment programmes for different groups in the adult population; and
- the provision of rehabilitation and other services for elderly and disabled people to maintain and restore their capacity for normal daily living.

Most countries of the Region now spend 3 – 10% of gross national product on health care, three quarters of which goes on hospital care. Advances in health technology now allow safe and efficient treatment of various conditions. Paradoxically, they have also contributed to an increase in the number of people requiring care and to the demand for rehabilitation and continuing care at home and in the community. Health care technology has been so successful that some countries overuse it while others, particularly in the central and eastern parts of the Region, experience acute shortages of basic drugs, vaccines and equipment. Serious efforts are being made to use health services more appropriately, taking account of the quality of life and the dignity of patients, particularly those who are seriously ill and dying, and emphasizing the quality of the care provided.

Primary health care is the foundation of appropriate care. Its position and importance have to be constantly restated to redress the balance weighted towards technological health care systems. Primary care is not the concern of general practitioners alone, but involves other professionals such as nurses, social workers and community-based pharmacists, who are equally important providers of health care and advisers on self-care.

A consideration of the full spectrum of disease – acute and chronic diseases, minor and major ailments – shows that health professionals provide only a part, albeit an extremely important one, of all personal health care. Most care is self-administered or provided by family members and friends. Yet individuals and families are seldom given sufficient information to make informed choices about the appropriate use of medical services or to participate equally with health professionals in making decisions. Many health care systems are not as sensitive as they should be to the needs of individuals and families, who as a result often make ineffective use of services.

The philosophy of health for all calls for better interaction, integration and coordination of services, for a multisectoral approach to prevention, health promotion, rehabilitation and care, and for formal recognition of the greater potential role of individuals, families and communities. Today, almost no country is fully satisfied with these aspects of its health services.

The new governments in the central and eastern parts of the Region face particular problems in reforming their health service systems in line with the pluralism of their political programmes. The demand for health services is likely to increase, owing to the backlog of unmet need, demographic trends, growing consumer expectations and technological progress. These countries also have to cope with problems related to health personnel, including demands for higher pay and the shortage of nurses and other professionals. Both governments and staff have to deal with change and uncertainty, as new funding mechanisms and organizational structures are introduced in the pluralist settings now developing in these countries.

The health service systems in all Member States are under increasing pressure to use all their resources efficiently, effectively and equitably. They are also expected to pay close attention to the satisfaction of both the general public and users with the services provided. The management has to be responsive to a health services workforce that expects fair rewards, both in comparison with the earnings of other occupational groups and as a recognition of the responsibilities and tasks it carries out. The workforce also expects good conditions of work, and the opportunity to carry out its tasks in ways that are professionally and personally satisfying.

These trends reinforce the need for comprehensive and linked information systems for all parts of the health service (community-based services, institutions and various agencies). These systems can track what is happening throughout the health service and provide timely, valid and relevant information for policy and operational decision-making. Such information systems must be very carefully designed to take into account concerns about ethics and confidentiality.

Both policy-makers and managers are under pressure to act on the most urgent day-to-day problems. If they understand the basic principles of health for all, it will give them a valuable strategic framework within which to make shorter-term decisions.

The need for greater equity in health requires forceful action to reduce the politically indefensible and socially unacceptable differences in access to services. These inequities can only be reduced by tackling the financial, cultural or physical barriers that limit access to appropriate care. Attention should also be paid to the unequal access that may result from decisions about resource allocation, funding mechanisms for services, and payment mechanisms for institutions and individual professional providers.

The principle of multisectoral collaboration also needs emphasis. Many patients' problems can only be addressed adequately if a number of sectors such as social welfare, housing and transport act jointly.

Accordingly, Chapter 6 has three groups of targets (see Fig. 5). The first group is concerned with the policies for health services (target 26) and their implementation through organization and management (target 27). Targets 28 – 30 focus on the three major types and settings of health care: primary health care in the community, hospital care as it supports primary care, and long-term care for the chronically ill and other groups with special needs. Target 31 explicitly addresses the quality and outcome of health care and technology.

Fig. 5. Appropriate care

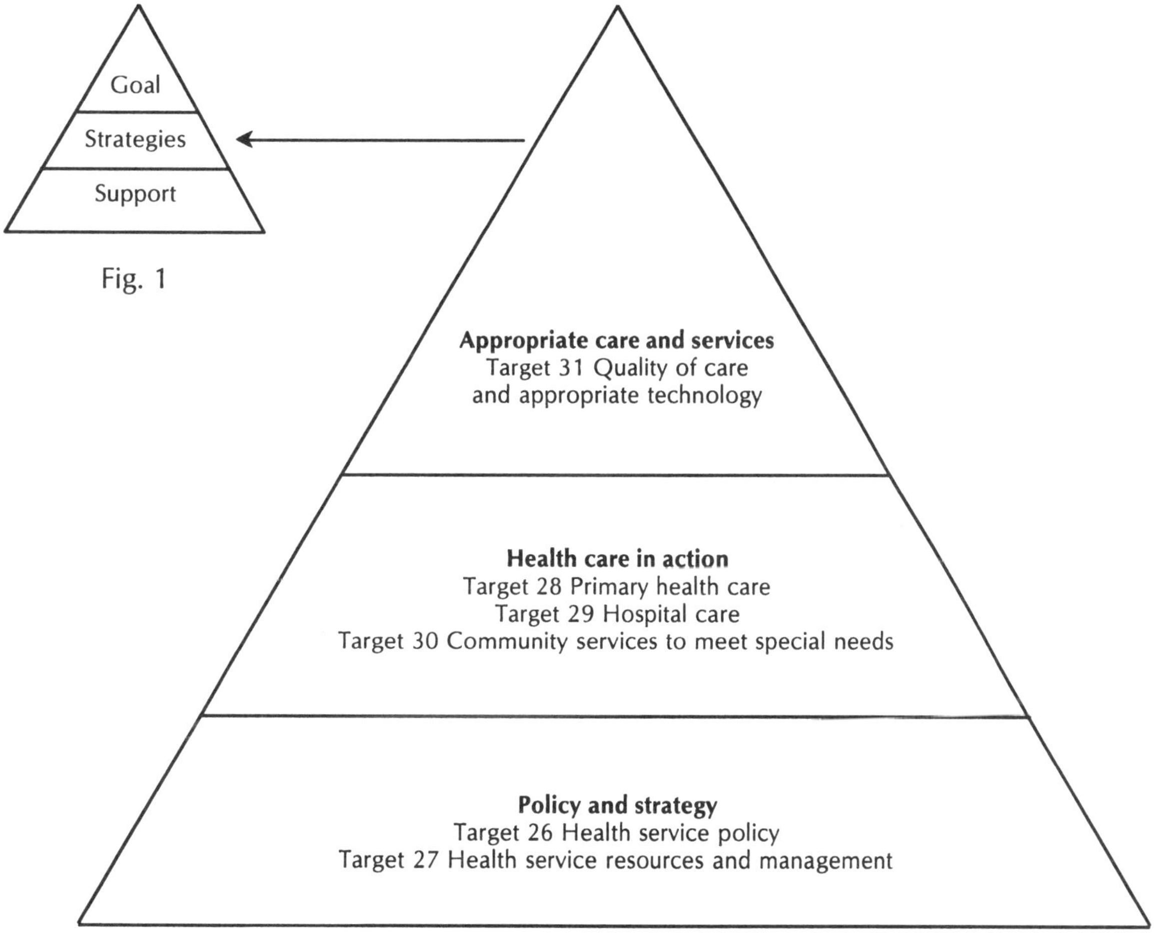

Goal

Strategies

Support

Fig. 1

Appropriate care and services
Target 31 Quality of care
and appropriate technology

Health care in action
Target 28 Primary health care
Target 29 Hospital care
Target 30 Community services to meet special needs

Policy and strategy
Target 26 Health service policy
Target 27 Health service resources and management

Target 26 – Health service policy

By the year 2000, all Member States should have developed, and be implementing, policies that ensure universal access to health services of quality, based on primary care and supported by secondary and tertiary care.

Achievement of this target will depend on the adoption, implementation and constant updating of clear-cut health service policies by appropriate bodies in all Member States, as an essential component of health for all policy. These policies should:

- *clearly state the lines along which health services will develop;*

- *be based on the principles of physical and economic accessibility, quality and cultural acceptability;*

- *establish primary care as the foundation for service delivery, supported by systems of secondary and tertiary care;*

- *make a commitment to continuing improvement in quality of care;*

- *secure the active participation of the public and health service providers in policy formulation and implementation.*

Problem statement   Most countries in the European Region have health service policies, but many of these policies have a very narrow focus, concentrating on organizational issues and the real but short-term needs of maintaining the infrastructure of current service provision. Few take a wider view that encompasses important components of health service policy, such as resources and management issues (see target 27) or the assurance of the quality of care and the use of appropriate technologies (see target 31).

Many policies claim to be set within the conceptual framework of health for all and acknowledge the principles of equity, accessibility and quality of care. Often, however, there are no mechanisms to ensure that these principles become a reality. The pursuit of productivity and efficiency, both laudable and necessary aims, has resulted in a preoccupation with political expediency, cost containment, the financing of services and the payment of health service providers *(1)*.

Health service policy often divorces the issue of health from the provision of services to deal with ill health. It is largely concerned with the more glamorous, high-profile technological services provided in modern hospitals. While these have an important part to play, an overall strategic direction is lacking. The long-term goal of improving the quality of care at all levels and the health of the population has been lost.

Health service policy is hard to realign to become an essential component of health for all strategies when clear developmental direction and guidance are missing. The principles of policy are simple to set out yet difficult to put into operation. They encompass accessibility and quality. They define primary and continuing care as the foundations of health service delivery, supported by secondary and tertiary services. They require improvements to the quality of all care and of specific technologies. They encourage the participation of health service providers and consumers in the formulation, development, implementation and evaluation of policy.

An equitable health service is without barriers to access for people in need. The organization of services can either limit or widen access. Currently, a number of physical, financial and cultural barriers block wider access to services in many parts of the Region. For example, health centres, doctors' premises, child health clinics and hospitals may be inconveniently located, incurring long, difficult or costly journeys. The times at which services are available may be inconvenient to patients, and language or cultural factors may inhibit communication between patients and health service personnel.

Until recently, the hospital was regarded as the basis of the health care system in almost every country in the Region. Today, many countries have policies that emphasize the central position of primary care, with services that are comprehensive and integrated, provided locally, organized intersectorally, and supported by secondary and tertiary services. Nevertheless, this is not always followed up with implementation strategies that promote primary health care. Too often the hospital sector receives the largest share of health care funding, while primary care services remain under-resourced. These services often include community nursing, homes for elderly people, home care services, and suitable care for people with mental disorders and for substance abusers. Many people who are most appropriately cared for in the community and who should receive primary care now fill hospital beds (2).

In most Member States, care providers contribute to policy formulation through their professional organizations. Such participatory mechanisms are just beginning to emerge in the central and eastern parts of the Region. These countries have traditionally taken a unified approach to policy on health services and the education of health professionals.

In many countries, efforts have been made to involve the public in policy formulation through community health councils, health insurance groups and elected bodies. Unfortunately, these activities have not always resulted in true participation, and need to be re-examined.

Suggested solutions   To develop health service policies as part of a wider health for all strategy, all Member States should review their existing policies and realign them to allow universal access to services of high quality. Establishing primary care as the cornerstone of health service policy would be a first step towards improving the quality of care. The commitment to quality should also apply to improvements in secondary care and participatory policy development and implementation.

Policies should have a clear strategic direction, while allowing flexibility and regular review as implementation develops. It would be unrealistic to expect one model policy for health services to be of use everywhere. Many systems operate in the Region at present. None are "pure" systems: no national health service is funded entirely from general taxation nor is any system based wholly on private insurance payments.

People should be clearly informed about the content of the care they can expect to obtain. They should know about the coverage of health needs, the functions and levels of care, the settings and types of health services and the standards of quality. There is a danger, however, of specifying too precisely what exactly a health service will do in the clinical arena. The policies most likely to succeed are those conceived and implemented with broad political, professional and public support in the voluntary, public and private sectors.

The means used to develop and act on agreed policy will vary according to circumstances. They typically include legislation and regulation to sustain the strategic intent: the designation of legal responsibilities for the delivery of health services, and the identification of functions and incentives for the coordination, control and provision of services. In addition, field experience and epidemiological studies have already proved useful in some countries by providing disaggregated small-area statistics that can help to identify local health needs.

Barriers to access can be tackled in many different ways. Policies on the financing mechanisms, ownership and functions of the provider institutions can be adjusted to ensure that people get the services they need when they need them. This means making basic health services available and accessible to people where they live and work, and reaching out to socially disadvantaged groups. It also means lowering

professional and social barriers between service providers and users, and improving communication with patients, self-help groups and social services.

Health care policy needs to ensure that services are comprehensive and coordinated. The whole resident population, including migrants, should have access to a full range of services that can improve their physical and mental health and rehabilitate those with physical, psychological and social disabilities. The services should actively address groups with specific health problems, including those needing long-term or terminal care.

Balancing primary health care with specialized care is an important task. Some countries have adopted the simple policy of devoting to primary health care any additional resources that become available.

Equally important is a policy focus on quality. All care provided, whether by first-contact services or after referral, should meet the individual's needs for care. Care should be humane, using procedures and technology of appropriate quality, and be provided by competent, trained staff. In addition, the care given should be a response to the individual's informed choice. To give care of high quality requires real commitment at all levels, from policy-makers through managers to staff delivering care.

A commitment to quality can be promoted through training at basic and postgraduate levels, through the accreditation of institutions, through the active involvement of the health professions in policy formulation, implementation and review, and through continuous learning from feedback on performance and outcomes.

Community groups, often in dialogue with health professionals, can address public and individual consumer satisfaction with, and confidence in, the quality and level of services provided. The community can help identify needs for expansion, reorientation or innovation in the health services. Policy should also address informal carers. They are an important health resource. They can work in partnership with voluntary services and health professionals to stimulate and support self-care and other forms of lay care. In addition, if community groups are involved they can help to educate the public in the informed and rational use of professional health services.

Target 27 – Health service resources and management

By the year 2000, health service systems in all Member States should be managed cost-effectively, with resources being distributed according to need.

This target can be achieved if:

- *management of health care systems and institutions is based on outcome targets for improved health and patient satisfaction;*

- *regionalization is adopted as a guiding principle in the allocation of resources to secondary and tertiary care;*

- *systems are established that facilitate distribution of resources according to community needs;*

- *financing and budgeting mechanisms support the cost-effective use of resources;*

- *the tasks of health care providers are appropriately defined to enable effective care to be dispensed in line with agreed policies and functions and to offer attractive conditions of employment;*

- *personnel management practices achieve teamwork, motivation, job satisfaction and the pursuit of excellence;*

- *information systems support planning and management based on health needs and cost-effectiveness.*

Problem statement Target 26 sets out the need for clear and well defined health service policies that operate within the framework of health for all. Target 27 tackles the issues of cost-effective management and an equitable distribution of resources based on population needs.

Organization Health services everywhere are under pressure because of the growth of technology and of people's needs and expectations. In addition, virtually all health service systems in the Region are experiencing financial difficulties. Many are undergoing organizational restructuring and introducing new management arrangements. These reforms often require radical change to rationalize decision-making and management operations and to review financing systems *(3,4)*.

A common problem, particularly in the central and eastern parts of the Region, is the assumption that change will quickly bring benefits. Furthermore, the financial costs of transition, the organizational disruption and the need to develop new management skills are often seriously underestimated. The management of change needs considerable support.

In some countries, the responsibility for health and health services is fragmented, while elsewhere it is fully centralized. In either case, there is often no incentive to meet the health needs of the population rather than the needs of organizational hierarchies and institutions. There are few clear, public and responsive health policies that describe targets, functions, settings and quality of care. The accountability for health outcome, performance and cost-effectiveness is often absent or diffuse.

Initiatives to reform the organization and management of health services have often been a piecemeal response to the immediate problems perceived by the government of the day. A long-term focus is usually lacking and management infrastructure is changed with little thought for the long-term consequences. Crisis management is not likely to meet targets for improving the health of the whole population or to satisfy patients. It defeats the objective of reorganization because it hinders the search for cost-effective solutions and thus prevents or delays the distribution of resources according to need.

Financing Many funding systems are in operation. Targets to reform systems of management and finance should not seek to be prescriptive, but should aim instead to provide a framework within which effective implementation of the current policy directions in each country can be maximized.

In some countries, reviews of financing mechanisms have resulted in proposals to shift the balance of service provision between the public and private sectors. Problems have often been tackled in isolation, such as the control of health service costs, the more effective use of resources, the reallocation of funds to agreed priorities for service development, or the adequate funding of essential services. A recurring problem is the difficulty of balancing the pressures of public policy outside the health sector, such as the containment of inflation and restraints on public expenditure, with those within the health system, such as the demands from care providers and consumers for better services, more modern technology and better care.

Experience with public and private funding has been varied. In the past decade, some countries have shifted towards public funding for health care systems, while others have moved towards private funding. Public sector funding, particularly where centrally controlled, can moderate health service costs and counteract inequities in access to care. Where governments do not give sufficiently high political priority to health, however, public funding may lead to serious and damaging underfunding, continuing inequities and a lack of incentives for efficient and effective service delivery and use. On the other hand, private sector funding can facilitate patient choice and provide physicians and other care providers with greater rewards for skill and effort. It does, however, risk increasing administration costs and may decrease the access disadvantaged people have to care. It can also encourage inappropriate treatment that is not relevant to patients' needs.

Service distribution   Health care resources include financial, staff and capital resources, such as buildings and technological equipment. The existing organization of these resources is not always rational or based on the needs of individuals or of the population.

Primary care is usually accessible to most of the population. It does not in all countries, however, serve as the means of entry into a health care system that truly identifies and meets needs. Some countries lack health professionals with the appropriate training, and others have too many in cities and too few elsewhere. Social service personnel, such as social workers and home helps, are often in short supply.

Secondary, usually hospital-based, care is often concentrated in the teaching hospitals of major cities. The hospital sector has often found it difficult to establish a rational countrywide network, organized to meet the needs of the population.

Personnel   The increased specialization of health workers, with the formal recognition of new professions, poses a formidable managerial challenge. While these developments have often improved particular aspects of patient care, they have also made it more difficult to match health workers to the functions and settings dictated by patients' needs. The result is that functions are often fragmented, especially the diagnosis, treatment and continuing care of the individual patient. Increased interprofessional teamwork is hard to achieve in the face of hierarchical practices. Providers' lack of motivation and cooperation has sometimes hampered the implementation of health service policies, because of inadequacies in communication, peer group support or incentives.

Outcome and performance   Changes in the financing of health services, ostensibly to redistribute resources according to need, have been closely allied to management reorganizations in many countries. Outcome and performance targets have rightly been espoused as the key to improving health, the treatment of ill health, the quality of health care and patient satisfaction.

Experience has revealed difficulties in using these measures because information is lacking and information systems for management decision-making are inadequate in areas such as the allocation and control of resources, service development, and the monitoring and evaluation of service outcomes.

Suggested solutions   The challenge is to organize and manage health service resources so that the policy objectives (universal access to health services, high quality of services, a focus on primary health care and better patient health and satisfaction) can be consistently met. Changes based on political ideologies must be set within this framework. They can still encompass a wide variety of choice in the exact balance of funding systems and in methods of managing health care and health care institutions.

Organization   The trend in several countries is towards the separation of financing and delivery, as in the United Kingdom, or towards multiple sources of funding as in France, Germany and the Netherlands. The disaggregation of rigidly hierarchical service structures into more autonomous or free-standing institutions is a feature of many countries in the central and eastern parts of the Region, while innovation has come from self-employed health care providers in Germany. A balance must be struck, however, between the decentralized provision of services and central direction, so that the overall policy objectives are not lost *(5 – 8)*.

Decentralization can also be achieved by devolution to regions, as in parts of Scandinavia. In a geographical region or district, primary care offices and facilities can be distributed to cover basic health needs at home and at work. At the same time, hospitals and other health services can be distributed to make up a service pyramid of different levels of specialization and catchment areas. The aim is to deliver the various components of service, such as prevention, diagnosis, treatment and rehabilitation, in the settings most appropriate to the needs of the patients. One interesting approach, used in a few pilot areas such as St Petersburg and on a more geographically widespread scale in the United Kingdom, has been to give primary health care providers funds with which to purchase secondary and other services on behalf of their patients *(8 – 10)*. This has the potential to ensure that all levels of service are responsive to needs, and that primary care forms the basis of health care delivery. On the other hand, such a high

degree of financial and management decentralization can also lead to uneven and unequally distributed care. Evaluation and accountability are very important, as has been demonstrated in Scandinavia. There, central health departments have the important functions of analysing the characteristics of their areas, defining the level and quality of services that a population needs, evaluating the meeting of basic functional needs in the area, and penalizing providers who do not meet required levels of coverage or standards of quality *(2)*.

Financing   Several countries have found it useful to review the balance of their public and private funding. Austria, particularly in the hospital sector, and Israel offer examples of the introduction of private business management and accounting methods into the health services. The recent health care reform in the Netherlands aims at universal coverage by insurance and a restructuring of the arrangements for financing and providing health care. Constant review is required to ensure that such methods indeed support health service efficiency and cost-effectiveness, while improving quality and accessibility. Routine outcome indicators, such as those produced in the United Kingdom, can be used for this purpose.

Any chosen form of health services financing (such as general taxation, national health insurance, compulsory employment-related health insurance, or the individual choice of a health insurance premium and benefits package) and resource allocation (such as budget and other forms of prospective allocation and reimbursement to institutions, agencies and providers) should ultimately ensure that each individual is entitled to and receives appropriate care. Devices such as out-of-pocket payments by patients, including co-payments and deductibles, as well as reimbursement mechanisms need to be very carefully constructed. They must ensure that their intended purpose of generating revenue or deterring unnecessary use does not prevent patients from seeking care when they need it. The danger is that the costs of collection may outweigh the income, especially for services with large numbers of exempted users.

Management All management arrangements should provide a framework in which agreed health service policies can be implemented. They should suit the general culture and organization of the country and ensure that the health care system as a whole functions smoothly and always in the interests of the patients rather than the providers. The arrangements should also ensure that individual institutions, agencies and providers are able to function effectively and efficiently with the resources available.

At the level of the health care institution, the manager's tasks are to set institutional objectives (within a framework of broader policies and objectives for the system as a whole), to identify the tasks that need to be carried out to harness the necessary resources (personnel, supplies, equipment and information) and to monitor activity and take corrective action when required. This implies a number of tasks such as personnel management (including the recruitment, training, development, retention and reward of staff), inventory management, internal maintenance of the building, and external relations with other institutions and the public.

Management should concentrate on outcomes and have explicit targets for policy objectives that include improving the health of the population and service delivery to individual patients. Monitoring and evaluating services against these targets and objectives is an important management function that will strengthen mechanisms for quality assurance. Regions, districts, institutions and individual providers have usefully compared their performance with that of their peers, for example in the United Kingdom *(11)*.

Personnel For performance to be measured fairly, tasks must be clearly defined and all staff must know what is expected of them. Salaries may or may not be linked to performance measures, but all payment systems should promote behaviour and activity that accords with policy intentions.

Effective personnel management requires an equitable policy for the remuneration of each category of health worker. This can be by salary or fee or in some other form, and can encompass other terms and conditions of contract, such as the type and level of responsibilities exercised, the expected hours of duty or availability, holiday entitlements, retirement benefits and opportunities for continuing education and professional development. With an equitable policy, each category of worker feels that the rewards and other conditions of work are fair.

One measure of high quality work is the cohesiveness of the whole health care system – the smoothness with which patients move through it and are served. Interdisciplinary teamwork is important so that family health physicians, nurses, social workers, physiotherapists, pharmacists and other professionals, each offering complementary skills, function together as a team, to provide a complete service to an individual patient, neighbourhood or group.

Information   Changes in health service financing and management require the support of well developed and integrated information systems. Data must be captured, ordered, linked, presented and interpreted in a way that makes them useful for planning, for clinical decision-making and for management.

The ideal, nowhere fully realized, is a shared information system that gives health care staff feedback on the efficiency, effectiveness and outcomes of their performance. Epidemiologists and health service planners can use such a system to identify the continuing and changing needs of the population served. They can also assess the cost-effectiveness and quality of the health service system. Senior managers can use it to monitor the allocation of resources among functions and client groups and to evaluate the efficiency, effectiveness and quality of the services provided. Policy-makers can link health service information with information from other sources to make strategic decisions on the future of health development. The aim is not one large database with free access to all, but rather a system of many databases that are linked while guaranteeing confidentiality and selectivity. Such systems are technically possible, but require careful design and development, backed up by training and support.

Target 28 – Primary health care

By the year 2000, primary health care in all Member States should meet the basic health needs of the population by providing a wide range of health-promotive, curative, rehabilitative and supportive services and by actively supporting self-help activities of individuals, families and groups.

This target can be achieved if Member States:

- *promote and provide preventive and curative health services, including diagnosis, treatment, care and rehabilitation, through locally organized delivery systems;*

- *provide community groups with technical, financial, information and other forms of support and make them active partners in the development of primary health care;*

- *remove all financial, physical and cultural barriers to the use of primary health care;*

- *strengthen active outreach to the community and cooperation with other sectors to achieve effective use of health services;*

- *ensure adequate numbers of appropriately qualified family health physicians and nurses for the primary health care services;*

- *organize primary care in such a way as to achieve integration of services based on teamwork among health care providers;*
- *ensure effective patient referral and the mutual provision of technical support by all levels of care.*

Problem statement   To meet the basic health care needs of the population, a wide range of services must be provided at a local level. These services need to be backed up by active support to individuals and community groups. The definition of "local" may vary according to the community, but access to primary health care services for all who need them is vital, as is outreach to the community and intersectoral collaboration.

All the countries in the European Region have the basic elements of a local primary health care system, although significant variations emerge in the range and level of services available locally to meet basic health needs. Even in the more prosperous countries of the Region, resources and services may be poorly distributed.

In reproductive and maternal health services, variations exist in quality, availability and accessibility. Antenatal and perinatal services exist everywhere, but their quality varies. The appropriateness of the technology used in the care of women before, during and after birth continues to be debated in some countries. Likewise, family planning and contraceptive services are not uniformly available. When termination of pregnancy is indicated on health grounds and is legally sanctioned, timely and appropriate services may not be available. In other cases, the health and social problems arising from the strict application of restrictive legislation on abortion, including the consequences of illegal abortions, may be underestimated. In addition, couples unable to conceive may not have access to

fertility clinics. Genetic counselling services are still unsatisfactory in some countries. People with sexual problems often have no access to appropriate counselling and treatment services.

In the field of child health services, immunization rates have shown a steady improvement in recent years. Important gaps in coverage persist, with some countries of the Region having particular problems *(12,13)*. The elimination of certain communicable diseases from the European Region (see target 5) will require more sustained cooperation from primary care workers, parents, community leaders and the public at large.

Outreach to the community is essential. In many areas of primary health care, the success of programmes depends on the cooperation and involvement of community groups as active partners in the development of appropriate and accessible services. A wide range of community groups caters for specific sectors of the population and offers opportunities to develop more effective and comprehensive services. Yet they are often an underused resource, operating in isolation from mainstream primary health care, and are not recognized and supported as active partners and co-workers. This partnership is particularly important when providing primary health care for groups of people with special needs (see target 30).

Primary health care services are not always well placed to support people coping alone or with the help of informal carers. Health care is not the sole prerogative of professionals, and many people cope on their own with a wide range of health problems. Many people find self-care attractive because it involves personal choice, and lets them control their bodies and make their own decisions.

Health workers have readily grasped the concept that primary health care is a professional service of first contact and the point of entry or referral to other levels of secondary and more specialized care. Primary health care includes not only family doctors, but also community-based nurses, health visitors, midwives and other health professionals such as speech therapists, chiropodists, psychiatric nurses, occupational therapists, dietitians and physiotherapists. These health professionals need to learn how to cooperate better with one another across disciplinary boundaries. They should be aware of each other's professional contribution, supplement each other's knowledge and skills, and make a broader contribution to the solution of complex problems facing individuals, families and communities.

In addition, health professionals need to work intersectorally with other providers such as social services and housing departments. In many countries, primary health care and related social services do not yet provide long-term follow-up for patients, after discharge from primary health care or hospital. Opportunities are lost for solving basic health problems effectively and for securing appropriate help from others for patients with psychological and social, as well as physical, problems. These issues become even more important with aging populations experiencing multiple difficulties.

One of the problems of ensuring integrated and continuing care is the increasing specialization of health professionals. The European Conference on Nursing in 1988 found that in some countries the shortage of nurses and the lack of well organized community and domiciliary nursing services reduce the possibility of providing a complete primary health care service *(14,15)*. In others, primary health care professionals lack the knowledge, skills and competence to coordinate care for their patients or clients in an effective way.

Continuity of care is essential and, while in all countries health services are operationally integrated through referral mechanisms, these mechanisms are not always well understood either by the general population seeking care or the people working in the services.

Suggested solutions   The basic values set out in the Declaration of Alma-Ata – such as the need for services to be available, culturally acceptable, affordable, accessible, and professionally and scientifically sound – remain valid and should continue to underpin the development of primary health care *(16 – 19)*.

Local, well integrated, community-based programmes addressing all aspects of primary health care need to be developed and supported. The changes and action needed to bring this about will vary from country to country according to the current situation. There is ample scope for supporting self-help and bringing together representatives of the community, the health services (particularly primary health care) and other sectors.

When radical change in the health service system is being contemplated, clear policies must be established, identifying the health objectives and contributions of the primary health care system. This process is by no means a simple one and no one system can be universally recommended. Primary health care can be realigned and tailored in many ways to the specific needs of the population it serves.

A searching review of existing practice is an essential first stage. This should clarify the nature and scale of actual and potential health problems. It should also estimate whether current diagnostic, therapeutic and rehabilitative care and outreach support really improve health and meet the needs of the patient. This will facilitate the development of policies that clearly state the range of services and technology required to meet the objectives, and the required numbers and abilities of the staff to be employed. The overall aim is to draw up policies that will bring about a real shift towards primary health care, and will ensure that patients are seen as a whole, in the context of their family circumstances and home and work environments.

The scope of activity for primary health care systems is broad. It includes disease prevention and control programmes, the use of clinical settings, home care and various media to educate the community about prevailing health problems, their effective prevention and control, and health promotion. It ensures the coordination and integration of care in an interdisciplinary and multisectoral way, where appropriate, and offers prompt, professionally sound treatment locally for conditions that do not require specialized attention. When necessary, the primary care worker arranges for the earliest possible referral to appropriate specialist providers and facilities.

Good primary care systems also value the patient's contributions to care. They encourage the participation of individuals and of self-help groups organized around specific health issues, such as those of diabetic patients and haemophiliacs' family organizations.

It is particularly helpful if families can have a close, long-term relationship with their own family physician and family nurse. Family physicians and nurses require a broad health for all outlook and a commitment to improving the quality of life of the people they serve. General practice is progressing towards this ideal. The concept of the health for all nurse has started to take root since the European Conference on Nursing in 1988. This basic health care worker provides, for a number of families and households, a continuous and integrated service of lifestyle counselling, home care and well-baby care.

Appropriate staff training is important and should include the development of skills that facilitate interdisciplinary teamwork, so that care can be closely coordinated and integrated to fit the individual patient's or client's needs. Changing a professional culture is a strategic task that will need to be addressed in both the basic and the continuing education of all health workers. Such education should encourage them to pursue excellence in their work and health for all values and objectives (see target 36).

Good primary health care professionals also act as advocates of the individual patient when in contact with the rest of the health service system. They communicate with lay people, recognize and effectively use the resources existing in the community, and integrate their activities with the skills and self-help efforts of individuals, families, carers and communities. Rules and conventions of practice on referral among primary health care providers and between them and secondary care providers should always operate in the patient's interest rather than for administrative or provider convenience.

Health administrators and managers must facilitate ready access to primary health care. Financing policies, usually set as part of a central policy, must not hinder the access of any individual or group to the services they need.

Target 29 – Hospital care

By the year 2000, hospitals in all Member States should be providing cost-effective secondary and tertiary care and contribute actively to improving health status and patient satisfaction.

This target can be achieved if hospitals:

- *actively support the provision of primary health care in the areas they serve;*

- *concentrate on specialized services requiring technology and skills that can be delivered efficiently only in institutional settings;*

- *assess their performance in terms of health status, quality of life, patient satisfaction and contribution to an improvement in community health;*

- *follow admission and discharge procedures that ensure effective links with primary health care and other community services, and strengthen information systems accordingly;*

- *ensure adequate numbers and an appropriate mix of health care providers and managers;*

- *organize care in such a way as to achieve integration of services based on teamwork among health care professionals;*

- *manage personnel, equipment, supplies and facilities cost-effectively.*

Problem statement   This century has seen a transformation in the role of hospitals. They are now placed at the very centre of medical science and technology. In recent decades, the resources allocated to health services have increased enormously throughout the European Region, especially those allocated to technological developments in medicine. These developments have led to more accurate diagnosis and effective treatment for a wide range of conditions. Some have enhanced the health, life expectancy and quality of life for patients, but few have greatly improved the health of the population as a whole *(20)*.

Technology has been increasingly emphasized, while the holistic nature of illness and thus the need to link hospital care with primary health care, particularly for rehabilitation and follow-up, have often been neglected. Hospitals have not usually attempted to assess their contribution to the health of the community they serve, or to monitor the effects of their activities on the health status, quality of life or satisfaction of individual patients. This has been due in part to inadequate information systems.

The scientific developments in hospitals have been accompanied by rising costs. These are exacerbated by public expectations of continuing medical innovation, by a growth in the range of services available and by a professional drive for excellence. Many technical innovations have been widely adopted, at great expense, without adequate evidence of their effectiveness. The challenge is to contain the consumption of costly resources while meeting patients' needs effectively, efficiently and appropriately, maintaining equity of treatment, respecting the ethics of patient care, and providing integrated services. Expensive services should no longer be offered when they have been shown not to benefit patients, so that resources can be spent instead on care of demonstrable value.

The trend towards specialized medical practice, dependent on technology, makes patient care complex and difficult to manage. Greater interdependence between clinical units makes it increasingly difficult to sustain the traditional culture of medical self-sufficiency and autonomy. Larger hospitals have often become difficult and stressful workplaces with high staff turnover. The culture of health professionals tends to favour trying to cope, rather than recognizing stress and seeking support.

Suggested solutions   Hospitals vary between countries. Many hospitals provide both inpatient and outpatient care, while others concentrate on inpatient care supplemented by ambulatory specialist practices. Countries in the central and eastern parts of the Region have inherited a hierarchical system of hospitals and polyclinics *(21)*. The

principles suggested here will need to be adapted to individual systems.

New role   The role of the hospital within the health service system as a whole needs to be adjusted. The aim is for hospital resources to be used to treat and care for people who need such highly specialized services, which can only be provided efficiently in an institutional setting. The high quality and cost-effectiveness of care are key objectives. Depending on the prevailing situation, such a reorientation may require legislative, economic, educational and other measures. France has adopted an innovative approach to this process through its comprehensive hospital law of July 1991 *(22)*.

In their new role, hospitals must put more emphasis on the continuity of care and coordinate their activities with long-term care services (see target 30) and with other primary health care facilities. They can actively support health promotion and primary health care in a number of ways. They can themselves provide settings for active health promotion. They can contribute to a healthy environment through well designed and implemented smoking, alcohol and nutrition policies and through proper waste management. They can support primary health care by sharing their diagnostic and therapeutic services (such as radiology, pathology, physiotherapy and occupational therapy) and by ensuring patients' access to primary health care on discharge. Hospitals have a traditional role as centres for research, innovation and the promotion of good practice. This can be extended to provide continuing education for primary health care staff, including joint reviews of cases and support for primary care research.

An international network of health-promoting hospitals has recently been initiated *(23)*.

Evaluation of care   To assess performance, the delivery of specialized services needs to be related to the health status and quality of life of individual patients. Performance can be measured only if clearly stated and well understood objectives have been set. If these are defined and quantified, they can form the basis for comparisons between institutions. Suitable indicators include readmission rates, complication rates, inappropriate admissions, waiting lists and waiting times, postoperative wound infection rates, contact with primary health care staff on a patient's discharge from hospital, and surveys of patient satisfaction. Since a hospital stay is usually only one of a number of episodes in the patient's journey through the health care system, hospital outcomes should ideally be related to the health of the patient over time, though inadequate information systems usually preclude this.

The evaluation of hospital care requires the investment of resources, time and effort into strengthening information systems, not only within hospitals themselves but at all levels of health care.

Staff issues   The deployment of hospital staff in primary health care settings allows the sharing of expertise and helps integration. In some places, hospital paediatric, psychiatric and geriatric staff assist primary health care staff in the assessment of needs and the continuing management of patients *(24)*.

Psychiatric nurses and other specialized hospital staff may be permanently attached to primary health care settings or be available to support the family by delivering hospital care at home. Some technical equipment can be used outside hospitals, allowing greater use to be made of outpatient and day-patient units, local and mobile clinics, and mobile teams of hospital personnel.

Conversely, there are also many examples of primary health care staff being based in or giving direct support to hospitals. This may include taking responsibility for patients in small long-term care facilities, such as local psychogeriatric units. Primary health care workers have great scope to serve as consultants, since they are familiar with the context of people's daily lives in which health problems arise.

Skilled staff working together in ways that maximize their effectiveness are an organization's most valuable asset. It is crucial to ensure that an appropriate number of staff is involved in management and in the direct provision of service, that all staff have the requisite competence for their tasks, and that a culture is fostered that promotes high quality care as well as cost-effectiveness. One important development, which must be further encouraged, is the greater readiness of staff to cooperate on an interdisciplinary level, to learn from others' experience and to be willing to compare their own work with that of colleagues.

Traditionally high-status staff, such as senior doctors, play a very important role in the deployment and use of resources and are often recognized as leaders in the local community. It is particularly important therefore that they acknowledge the need for change and set an example of how to function in a new managerial culture.

Management   The new role of hospitals requires a new style of management and a new sense of direction within the overall health care system. All hospital staff can practise innovative teamwork and show greater accountability with the help of information systems that focus on groups of patients and link clinical data with information on outcomes, resource use and costs.

Hospitals are not only places for diagnosis, treatment and care, but also complex economic organisms. A number of countries have recently tried to transform the business role of the hospital by creating market models that separate the planning and purchasing functions from the provision of services function *(25,26)*. This means that services are offered to purchasers at a specified price that reflects cost. The system is intended to promote competition between institutions and make comparison between them normal practice. Such a system requires a new type of manager, who is professionally trained both in business administration and in the health and hospital fields, and who can mobilize hospital units to cooperate to reach a common goal. In many instances, these functions will be shared among several managers. An important task for these managers will be to monitor the degree to which a more market-oriented approach (or, indeed, any management approach) encourages hospitals to deploy personnel, equipment, supplies and information in ways that enhance the quality of care and optimize their contribution to the health of the population.

Target 30 – Community services to meet special needs

By the year 2000, people in all Member States needing long-term care and support should have access to appropriate services of a high quality.

This target can be achieved if in all Member States country, regional and local authorities:

- *develop health care services specifically designed to meet the special needs of people suffering from chronic illness or from physical, mental or social disability;*

- *coordinate health services with social and income support services and establish appropriate communication;*

- *provide self-help and similar groups with support and facilitate their active participation in service planning and delivery;*

- *make arrangements to ensure access to high-quality care and support, including effective outreach services, and to monitor the continuity and quality of care.*

Problem statement   Every Member State has groups of people with long-term health care needs. They require services especially tailored to their circumstances, if they are to live as full and independent lives as possible. These groups include people of all ages who suffer from chronic conditions such as cardiovascular disease, cancer, diabetes and musculoskeletal disorders. They also include people with learning difficulties, those who have been physically disabled from birth or because of injuries, and those with chronic mental illnesses. Some of these conditions are more common in the less advantaged social groups. Typically, the average (healthy) life span differs by five to six years between the highest and lowest social classes. Even the most affluent countries of the Region show a three- to fourfold social class difference in rates of disability and chronic pain.

The "greying" of Europe is another important factor. By the year 2000, the Region will have almost 70 million people aged 70 years and over, compared with around 60 million in 1980. A number of people this age suffer from the degenerative diseases of old age, as well as from social isolation, and they are often less likely, and less able, to seek professional assistance.

Terminally ill people pose special ethical and practical problems. Too often, high-technology care is used in an effort to prolong life, when in fact it reduces the quality of the life remaining to patients and prevents them from dying with dignity in a situation of their choice.

Moreover, appropriate social support for these "Cinderella" groups – frail elderly, disabled and terminally ill people – is often lacking. Home services are often underfunded and many elderly people are misplaced and unsupported in long-term hospitals or nursing homes of low quality. Elderly and disabled people who have maintained some degree of independence in their own homes often lack essential clinical and social services that could correct their eyesight, assist their hearing and mobility, and provide them with home help and home nursing. For example, in some countries there are long waiting lists for hip replacement operations that could enable elderly people to recover their mobility and live more satisfying lives.

The very success of health promotion and disease prevention increases the demands on nursing and other caring services for these vulnerable groups. Their needs are not automatically met by the normal routines of primary health care or referral to secondary and tertiary services. They may not be covered adequately by the health insurance systems. The medical orientation and organization of health care often causes home care services, nursing homes and other support programmes to lack influential sponsors and advocates. They are therefore underfunded and slow to develop. This has been especially true of social work and housing adaptation, which fall outside mainstream medical care.

Special needs often call for complex solutions. They require continuity of care rather than a single professional provider acting autonomously and applying only one narrow range of technology or treatment.

A major challenge is to harness the contribution of other sectors, notably social services, housing and transport. The problem is not always a shortage of facilities or personnel, but a lack of communication, cooperation and coordination among the various sectors.

Self-help activities also need support. Care has generally come to be seen as the prerogative of professionals, yet individuals and families cope with a wide range of health problems. Such tasks often place heavy demands on the informal carers, but they may find it difficult or impossible to participate in major decision-making processes. Professionals, planners and politicians make choices on behalf of people with special needs and their carers, without consulting them on what is really needed, wanted, acceptable or useful.

Suggested solutions The prevention of illness and handicap is an important aspect of community services. As part of primary health care, it should focus on healthy elderly people and on those in poor socioeconomic circumstances, such as people who are single and homeless or long-term unemployed, to prevent them from becoming chronically ill.

The basic approach should be to develop well integrated, community-based programmes. These should be part of the primary health care function but sufficiently flexible to be specifically tailored to the circumstances and requirements of individuals with long-term and other special needs.

Long-term disabled people Care programmes for people with long-term needs, such as those who are chronically ill, severely disabled or frail and elderly, should be planned, developed and organized in partnership with the people needing the services. The aim should be to maximize their capacity to live an independent and fulfilling life.

Much more could be done to help disabled people to function independently in the community, by relatively simple modifications of dwellings and public buildings, and by specially adapted local public transport. New technology in the expanding field of human performance engineering, such as the "stand-up" wheelchair, can make highly significant improvements to the quality of life and functional ability. In addition, people with psychological or emotional problems can benefit from housing that is conducive to social contact and community cohesion.

Terminally ill people The care of terminally ill people has improved greatly with the development of the hospice movement, which has helped to define their special needs. The quality of life of terminally ill people reflects the quality of the support they are given by professional care providers and family members or other informal carers. This quality can be judged by how well their symptoms are controlled and their mental alertness is maintained, and by their ability to participate in daily activities and maintain social contacts, with assistance if necessary. The aim is for these patients to be able to make active use of their time during the working day, gain personal satisfaction out of the way that time is used, retain an interest in the world outside and maintain a sense of hope and something to live for. The health care and social support services should ensure that everyone who works with terminally ill people acquires these values and the skills to act on them.

Training Serving people with all types of special need requires a shift in attitudes and working methods. Health care professionals should, through training and continuing education, gain a broader understanding both of patients' needs and of the contributions of other professionals. They have to acquire the ability to manage multiple and complex problems. Senior personnel in professions such as nursing and social work should be more directly involved in medical education at all levels. This should include practical training in teamwork, so that they can complement the knowledge and skills of other team members, and make a specific contribution to meeting the special needs of individuals and families.

Resources   Support services and financial assistance from sectors other than health can be used to allow disabled or frail people to live close to their families in their own communities. Support for self-care, self-management (particularly within the family) and other services outside the health sector can be strengthened. For example, lay people, particularly those with complex problems, can be trained to handle their health problems, take preventive measures, recognize symptoms that need professional help, and understand the availability of, access to and appropriate use of various services. Professionals must recognize how much individuals do and how effective it often is. They should consciously engage the individual, the family and other carers in the management of problems.

Monitoring   A systematic review of services can help to assess their effectiveness and the quality of the care given. It can also point to the organization and managerial responsibility most conducive to effective action. Programme indicators are particularly useful for measuring the services provided and their outcomes, the degree of teamwork among different care providers, the effectiveness of the services for people who need long-term care and the satisfaction of the people using them.

Target 31 – Quality of care and appropriate technology

By the year 2000, there should be structures and processes in all Member States to ensure continuous improvement in the quality of health care and appropriate development and use of health technologies.

This target can be achieved through:

- *combined strategies for the assessment and promotion of the quality of care, the selection, development and proper use of appropriate technology, and the training of personnel;*

- *international collaboration and information exchange on assessment procedures, care standards, training and technology development.*

Maintaining the quality of care requires:

- *systematic monitoring of outcomes of health, quality of life, patient satisfaction, cost and affordability, based on appropriate information systems;*

- *use of appropriate incentive systems based on the outcomes of care, including feedback of comparable information on outcomes to individual providers and managers and to consumers;*

- *reorientation of the training of health service personnel to strengthen the emphasis on health status, quality of life, patient satisfaction and cost-effectiveness as perform-ance measures.*

Achieving the development and proper use of appropriate technologies requires:

- *building effective procedures for assessing benefit and appropriateness into the development of equipment, pharmaceuticals and other supplies and into their routine use throughout the health care system;*

- *monitoring of adverse effects to avoid the continued use of harmful or inappropri-ate technology.*

Problem statement Good quality of care means that individuals, families and communities receive care that is sensitive to their needs, acceptable to them and provided in the most appropriate setting (primary health care, hospital care, long-term care or home care). Quality development is an important policy aim in target 26. Good quality enhances the cost-effectiveness of care (target 27), and it measures the success of care in targets 28 to 30. Thus, quality assurance and development are an overall umbrella for Chapter 6.

The quality of care currently varies within and between countries and among service providers. This is partly because of the way health care is organized and practised, and partly because the structures and processes for ensuring quality contain weaknesses. A further problem is the very small share of health care resources devoted to the assessment and assurance of quality *(27).*

More fundamentally, most of the existing mechanisms used to ensure quality do not give health care providers any incentives to change practice, nor do they allow consumers to have a voice. Without a system that informs health care providers about the practices and outcomes of their peers, in other institutions and geographical areas, professional interest in quality issues is difficult to stimulate.

Information abounds on how health care is provided, but it tends to concentrate on measures of input and process rather than outcome, such as health improvement, quality of life, patient satisfaction and cost-effectiveness. It also tends to focus on individual patients, procedures and utilization, while data linkage is often hampered for reasons of confidentiality. Many quality assurance projects have been undertaken in isolation by individuals or individual clinical teams. In most instances, a piecemeal approach is also perpetuated by the lack of agreed professional strategies, including quality standards, indicators and information support.

Good care incorporates quality assurance and development. This message is not sufficiently emphasized during training, however, so many health providers resist the idea of the routine, systematic monitoring of quality, wrongly arguing that this would mean diverting time and resources from health care.

Development and availability of technology

Technology by the usual definition covers equipment, machinery, medical supplies and substances (including pharmaceuticals) and other supplies used in patient care. In a wider sense, technology is a whole range of facilities including not only the hardware (equipment, drugs and other supplies) but also health care procedures and the organization of patient care.

By either definition, technology is a means of delivering health care services; it is not an end in itself. Assessment therefore does not mean primarily appraising an individual piece of equipment, a drug or a procedure in a laboratory setting to judge its mechanical functioning, safety and efficacy. Evaluating the contribution a given technology makes to the quality of care provided is more important. Particular procedures, users of equipment and supplies may sometimes be so essential for the quality of care that they can serve as "tracers" of quality. More often, quality will depend on the interplay of a number of different technologies and factors.

In recent years, the development of new technologies has progressed rapidly, raising questions of affordability. Progress has not been even throughout the Region, resulting in wide differences in access to equipment and devices and in the availability of pharmaceuticals and supplies. It is particularly worrying that, in some countries, obsolete technologies are still used (28).

The countries of the central and eastern parts of the Region present special problems. In many cases, health service equipment and pharmaceutical industries have been dismantled as part of rapid economic change. Several countries have major gaps in specific types of technology, such as aids for people with disabilities. These countries often find imported technology too expensive to purchase in the appropriate quantities, with the result that they suffer severe shortages of basic equipment, drugs and vaccines. Where equipment is available, the problem is often the incompatibility between different types of technology and the lack of spare parts (29).

In the European Region, pharmaceuticals tend to be more strictly and stringently regulated than are equipment and other supplies. All countries have some system of licensing and procedures to control the marketing of drugs, but standards vary throughout the Region. In countries with sizeable industries that produce equipment, pharmaceuticals and medical supplies, export and employment interests also play a role in decision-making. More fundamentally, many providers as well as the general public believe mistakenly that "high-tech" processes are themselves direct indications of good quality of care.

Producers and regulatory agencies are responsible for the assessment of new technologies. Little feedback has come from health care practitioners or the public. Comprehensive assessment and monitoring systems have therefore been difficult to institute.

The assessment of pharmaceuticals and equipment has often been divorced from everyday practice. It tends to concentrate on easily measured factors such as safety, efficacy and cost and to make narrow assumptions about the use of technology. For example, testing a drug for a specific clinical purpose, within a defined protocol using randomized controls, becomes less relevant when the drug is used in the field for quite different conditions. The experts who assess the selection, development and dissemination of technology rarely have sufficiently broad training and education to take account of the everyday uses, procedures and organizational arrangements for the drugs, equipment and supplies in question.

Use of technology   In health care delivery, the use of technology is rarely assessed on a routine basis. Long-established products and processes are rarely evaluated, and assessment is particularly uncommon in primary health care. Institutional and disciplinary barriers and lack of expertise in assessment combine to hamper progress.

Health care providers need to concentrate on the comprehensiveness and continuity of care, rather than on individual items of technology. They have difficulty in recognizing how technologies combine to affect the quality of the care they deliver. In addition, a single provider may not have a sufficient number of cases and services to draw statistically relevant conclusions about quality.

Most providers of care do not collect adequate data to analyse and monitor their services. This means it is difficult to weigh objectively actual and commercially claimed benefits. Lack of appropriate information makes it difficult for providers and consumers to learn from practice and adjust their behaviour accordingly.

An additional danger is that the choice between alternative technologies is based on the preferences of individual providers and managers, rather than on a strategic assessment of their quality, effectiveness as treatment, patient satisfaction, and cost. For example, end-stage renal failure may be treated by different regimens of transplantation and dialysis. Even where a strategic assessment leads to the choice of transplantation, however, it may still not address all the issues such as the availability of donors, access to appropriate hospital and community services, and the resulting quality of life.

All countries have systems that monitor the adverse effects of drugs, based on reporting by individual doctors on their own initiative. Improvements are needed, however, to induce a wider response, to spot the harmful effects of drug interaction that affect special groups such as elderly people, and to provide feedback to those collecting the data. Most of the systems in operation fail to inform users about the findings, making it difficult to induce them to change their practice. The systems should not only alert practitioners about harmful effects but also identify shifts in indications, use, practice and health outcomes.

Suggested solutions   Health administrations, associations of providers and others involved in health care must have clear strategies and programmes on quality and technology development in health care. They should address the different responsibilities of each level of care. In so doing, they should clarify the process of assessment to be used, the results they expect and their consequences for health care practice. Strategies and programmes will have to be formulated very carefully so as to facilitate the purposeful involvement and cooperation of provider groups, researchers, policy-makers at different levels, public health authorities and consumers. Specific efforts, including appropriate training, will be required to make it clear that quality development is a responsibility that all must share.

An important part of the strategy is to have an information system that continuously focuses on the outcomes, achievements and cost-effectiveness of care; identifies the best achievers; looks at their practice, innovations and use of technology; indicates the important elements and characteristics underlying their success; and builds on professional pride and ethics to motivate providers to measure, discuss and constantly improve the quality of their care.

Motivation   The most powerful incentive for change is the sharing of information on the quality of care and the appropriateness of technology. Authorities should support meetings between health care providers, health administrations and authorities, patients, consumer groups, industry and research institutes. At national and other levels, steps can be taken to disseminate examples of good practice and innovative information tools. Quality development is a dynamic process that goes beyond conventional mechanisms, such as certification, licensing, standard setting and review, and compulsory medical audit, which by themselves provide insufficient incentives for change.

One of the most important steps in quality development is to motivate health care providers to take a critical look at the quality of their care. At least one approach has been shown to improve quality: the comparison of practice, utilization and cost in relation to outcome, for specific health problems, conditions or diseases.

Giving comparative information to individual care providers and units about their performance is a powerful means of self-improvement. It is a basis for both individual and collective learning, especially about methods and approaches that have proved to be helpful and have demonstrated good quality and improved health.

Development and dissemination   Policies on health technology in Member States should include the adoption and dissemination of technologies. They should also include mechanisms to review the effectiveness of particular diagnostic, therapeutic and rehabilitative technologies. The development and dissemination of technology require a mix of incentives and regulations, depending on the particular circumstances of each country. The most important factor is to improve the input from health care practice. Assessment needs to be carried out in routine clinical settings rather than under laboratory conditions.

A comprehensive policy for pharmaceuticals addresses drug legislation and registration, quality assurance, pricing, drug supply, drug information, drug utilization, education in the prescribing and use of drugs, and drug research and development. Such a policy would ensure the adequate supply of safe and effective drugs of good quality at a reasonable price and their appropriate use.

Policies in countries can go a long way towards giving strategic direction to the development of technology and quality. Policy-makers may, for example, promote research priorities in relatively neglected areas, encourage the judicious use of economic instruments, strengthen safety regulations, formulate policies on the promotion and advertising of technologies and promote industry's cooperation with health authorities, care providers, hospital managers and research institutes.

Assessment of outcome   The assessment of the quality of care and the appropriateness of technology share the same criteria of success: outcomes. This points to the usefulness, at all levels, of a routine assessment of outcomes such as better patient care, health outcomes, patient satisfaction and overall quality of life. This process requires the development and use of clear outcome indicators. Ethical issues should always be taken into consideration, to ensure that implementing the proposed strategies improves health, equity and the acceptability of care. The constraints of available resources should always be borne in mind.

When new technologies are being developed, clear assessment criteria should be applied. It may be helpful to ask such questions as: Will this new technology significantly improve health? Does it make existing technology obsolete? Is it cost-effective when used throughout the system? Will it make care less painful or more acceptable to the patient?

Monitoring of effectiveness   For economic and practical reasons not all technologies can be under scrutiny simultaneously. The first technologies to be assessed might be those that have potentially high risks, are expensive or are most commonly used. It is particularly important to monitor any adverse effects that could render the continued use of a technology inappropriate. Policies, legislation, regulations and practices should indicate clearly what action should be taken if the technology is found to be inappropriate or ineffective.

For example, formal mechanisms are needed to make systematic and proper evaluations of drugs before and after marketing, and to make accurate and complete information about drugs and their proper use easily available to health professionals and the public. Continuous follow-up of their use in clinical practice is also needed to assess their effects and side effects.

Feedback from practice   Information systems for the development of quality and technology must systematically monitor actual practice and resulting changes in health status, quality of life, patient satisfaction with care received, and costs. As this list indicates, different types of data need to be brought together from many provider institutions, professional disciplines and locations, as well as from patients and industry, while safeguarding their confidentiality. Such an information system can help to pinpoint the procedures and technologies that are most crucial for quality development. Where this has been done, as in the case of diabetes, monitoring can focus on these critical indicators, thus simplifying the process of data collection and analysis. Professional organizations should be encouraged to develop a consensus on quality indicators that they can accept and use effectively for the practical monitoring and assessment of technologies.

Some countries have found it useful to obtain input from the users of health care. They may be asked about their perceived health status before, during and after treatment, the changes in the quality of their lives, and the level of their satisfaction with the content and amenities of care and with the attention they receive. There is ample scope for surveys once a period of care is over, such as on discharge from hospital. Users may be more interested in providing information before and during care, if they can thereby influence the process and outcome of the care. They may, however, be inhibited if they are not convinced that their responses will be kept confidential and fear that criticism may adversely influence their care.

Education and training   The training of all health staff, as well as staff in other sectors, should particularly include quality development, as well as methods for the assessment and use of health care technology.

Progress has been made in some countries by disseminating information to the general public more effectively and by consulting consumer interest groups on a continuing basis, to agree on appropriate expectations of quality.

International collaboration   International collaboration has ample scope for sharing ideas and information and pooling comparative data. International work can also help develop acceptable care standards and training programmes. Since the scope of technology assessment is already too vast for many countries to deal with on their own, it is particularly suited to international action. International solidarity can also help alleviate the acute drug, vaccine and equipment shortages in the central and eastern parts of the Region and help these countries develop and modernize appropriate industries in this field.

References

1. *Health dimensions of economic reform*. Geneva, World Health Organization, 1992.

2. MILLS, A. ET AL., ED. *Health system decentralization: concepts, issues and country experience*. Geneva, World Health Organization, 1990.

3. ARTUNDO, C. ET AL., ED. *Health care reforms in Europe*. Proceedings of the first meeting of the Working Party. Copenhagen, WHO Regional Office for Europe, 1993 (document EUR/ICP/PHC 210(B)).

4. *Planning and management for health*: report on a European Conference. Copenhagen, WHO Regional Office for Europe, 1986 (EURO Reports and Studies, No. 102).

5. *Care in the Netherlands 1992. A summary of the financial overview of the care sector 1992*. Rijswijk, Ministry of Welfare, Health and Cultural Affairs, 1992 (document).

6. *Choices in health care*. A report by the Government Committee on Choices in Health Care. Rijswijk, Ministry of Welfare, Health and Cultural Affairs, 1992.

7. *Crossroads. Future options for Swedish health care*. Stockholm, Federation of Swedish County Councils, 1991.

8. *The health of the nation. Summary of the strategy for health in England*. London, H.M. Stationery Office, 1992.

9. HÅKANSSON, S. ET AL. *Leningrad revisited*: report of a second visit to the USSR, October 1989. Copenhagen, WHO Regional Office for Europe, 1990 (document SSR/MPN 501).

10. *Organization and financing of health care reform in countries of central and eastern Europe*: report of a meeting. Geneva, World Health Organization, 1991 (document WHO/DGO/91.1).

11. ÖVRETVEIT, J. *Health service quality. An introduction to quality methods for health services*. Oxford, Blackwell Scientific Publications, 1992.

12. *Fourth European meeting of national pro-gramme managers on the Expanded Programme on Immunization*: report on a WHO meeting. Copenhagen, WHO Regional Office for Europe, 1992 (document EUR/ICP/EPI 027).

13. *Expanded Programme on Immunization*: report of the 14th Global Advisory Group. Geneva, World Health Organization, 1992 (document WHO/EPI/GEN/92.1).

14. *European Conference on Nursing*: report on a WHO meeting. Copenhagen, WHO Regional Office for Europe, 1989.

15. *Health for all: the nursing mandate*. Copenhagen, WHO Regional Office for Europe, 1991 (Health for all nursing series, No. 1; document EUR/ICP/HSR 339).

16. *Alma-Ata 1978. Primary health care*. Report of the International Conference on Primary Health Care, Alma-Ata, USSR, 6 – 12 September 1978. Geneva, World Health Organization, 1978 ("Health for All" Series, No. 1).

17. *Needs assessment in local areas and its conse-quences for health care provision*: report on a WHO meeting. Copenhagen, WHO Regional Office for Europe, 1993 (document EUR/ICP/PHC 340).

18. *Continuity of care in changing health care systems*: report on a WHO Working Group. Copenhagen, WHO Regional Office for Europe, 1992 (document EUR/ICP/PHC 344).

19. *The role of primary health care in changing lifestyles*: report on a WHO Working Group. Copenhagen, WHO Regional Office for Europe, 1989 (document EUR/ICP/PHC 331).

20. JÖNSSON, B. ET AL, ED. *Policy making in health care – changing goals and new tools*. Lin-köping, WHO Collaborating Centre, 1990 (Health Service Studies, No. 4).

21. *Analysis of the organization of hospitals and health institutions at the district and community level in CMEA countries*: report on a study. Copenhagen, WHO Regional Office for Europe, 1990 (document EUR/ICP/PHC 644).

22. VANG, J. & WENNSTRÖM, G., ED. *Health care systems at the crossroads*. Linköping, WHO Collaborating Centre, 1991 (Health Service Studies, No. 6).

23. *Hospitals and health – networking into the future*: report on a WHO Workshop. Copen-hagen, WHO Regional Office for Europe, 1992 (document EUR/ICP/PHC 646(1)).

24. *Quality development in nursing care: from practice to science*: report on a WHO meeting. Copenhagen, WHO Regional Office for Europe, 1992 (document EUR/ICP/PHC 645).

25. *The role of hospitals in meeting the demands of an aging population: management policies*: report on a WHO Working Group. Copen-hagen, WHO Regional Office for Europe, 1990 (document EUR/ICP/PHC 631).

26. KOGEUS, K., ED. *The response of hospitals to the changing needs of the population*: report on a study. Stockholm, Swedish Planning and Rationalization Institute for Health and Social Services (SPRI), 1990.

27. BROOK, R.H. ET AL. Geographic variations in use of services: do they have any clinical signifi-cance? *Health affairs*, **3**(4): 63 – 73 (1984).

28. VANG, J. Technology assessment and primary health care in Europe. Issues and problems. *International journal of technology assess-ment in health care*, **5**: 111 – 119 (1989).

29. RACOVEANU, N.T. A WHO training package aimed at improving the use of radiology for underserved populations. *WHO chronicle*, **40**: 135 – 140 (1986).

7

Health for all development strategies

The factors contributing to the achievement of better health lie outside as well as within the health sector. The principles and strategies of health for all must therefore gain wide political acceptance in the European Region. This will also promote a greater commitment to implementation. Progress towards the health for all goals will take place in a climate of opportunity, but also of uncertainty.

The complexity and difficulty of making wise spending choices are likely to increase. As political, business and other decision-makers gain a better understanding of the contribution that health protection and promotion strategies could make to the achievement of their own objectives, they will realize the need to invest in health. Advances in health care technology and the aging of the population will boost demand for greater expenditure on medical and nursing services. While many politicians see this growth in expenditure as unsustainable, the basic principle of equity demands that people with similar or comparable needs have equal access to care (1). Ethically, this right cannot be jettisoned in the interests of cost containment or a balanced budget. Economists and other policy analysts should find ways of resolving this dilemma, and provide guidance in choosing between alternative ways of using resources.

Leadership: meeting the challenges Creative and flexible leadership will be essential to carry the health systems of the Region through this period of transition. Such leadership will be found in political, managerial and professional spheres. It must maintain the political visibility of health in countries and international bodies. It must sustain health workers' confidence and attract support from those outside the health sector who are crucial to the achievement of better health. It must also continue to promote innovation and quality in treatment and care. At the same time, the political, economic and social changes taking place throughout the Region, particularly in the central and eastern part, should make it possible to experiment with and develop new policies and structures to protect and promote public health. These changes should also allow new forms of organization to evolve that will be more effective in meeting the health care needs of the population.

The achievement of health for all depends on effective measures to secure greater equity in health, to promote healthy lifestyles, to create environments that sustain good health and to ensure access to appropriate care. Each of these policies and related actions presents a number of important challenges.

For example, achieving equity in health and better access to the prerequisites for health may involve re-examining the aims and priorities of overall social policy. Health promotion emphasizes the importance of public policy in creating social and physical environments conducive to healthy living. The development of settings for healthy living takes account of the social as well as the physical environment, and also calls for new structures and processes to facilitate community participation. Environmental health stresses not only better control of air, water and soil pollution and waste disposal, but also living and working environments that protect and maintain good health. Preventing pollution requires systems of planning and decision-making that work across the departmental lines of the public sector at all levels. It also depends on cooperation between the public, private and voluntary sectors. The focus on appropriate care reflects the continuing movement towards primary care and the prevention of disease and disability, coupled with efforts to improve the quality of life, particularly for those who are chronically ill. Strengthening teamwork in primary care and disease prevention requires not just new forms of health care organization but a different emphasis in professional education.

Health for all development means providing support to ensure that these challenges can be met. Health for all broadens the definition of health policy and strategy. It creates a new emphasis on public health that asserts the importance of community involvement and the contribution to health objectives that other sectors can make.

The targets in this chapter address the basic needs that must be met for sound health for all development: the development of knowledge and information support for policy and action; the creation of the requisite managerial infrastructures; the development of human resources for health; the mobilization of resources and broad social support; and the advocacy and practice of ethical values (Fig. 6).

Formulating policy   Policy is the foundation of health for all development. Target 33 defines the characteristics of such policies as reflecting the fundamental principles of reducing inequities, promoting health, preventing disease and disability and providing appropriate care. The challenge of creating opportunities for healthy patterns of living and for healthier environments, and the task of ensuring equitable access to health services together require the achievement of comprehensive and balanced policies, as called for in target 33. The challenge for the 1990s is to translate promises into practice in a way that matches the progress in policy adoption in the past decade.

Resources for health for all development   Research strategies and information systems are important sources of the knowledge required to support health for all development. Targets 32 and 35 are concerned with the acquisition of the knowledge needed to evaluate present policy and practice, to plan for the future and to make management decisions. The challenge for research is to develop programmes that will address the practical questions emerging in health for all development.

Fig. 6. Health for all development strategies

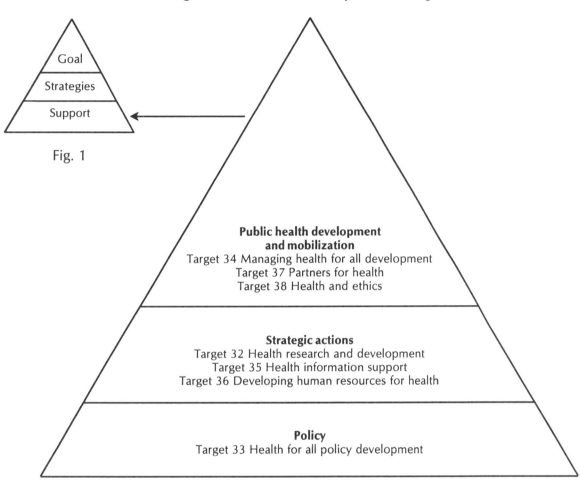

Fig. 1

**Public health development
and mobilization**
Target 34 Managing health for all development
Target 37 Partners for health
Target 38 Health and ethics

Strategic actions
Target 32 Health research and development
Target 35 Health information support
Target 36 Developing human resources for health

Policy
Target 33 Health for all policy development

Information needs are many and varied, arising in situations extending from medical practice to strategic choice. Information systems must develop in ways that make them relevant and accessible to the user. Their importance reflects the fact that health for all development is occurring in an information society. Information of all kinds, analysed and presented in appropriate formats, can do much to establish a foundation for effective cooperation between sectors.

The health system, as visualized in health for all, requires properly trained, professionally competent workers. Health care management requires stronger teamwork, a more effective use of personnel and the provision of work environments that support high quality care. Nevertheless, many of the people who can contribute to health for all work outside the health care sector: in education, environment, agriculture, architecture, urban planning and elsewhere. One of the greatest challenges of this decade is to influence the education and training of workers in sectors other than health, so that they support and reflect health for all values and objectives more widely in their professional practice. Target 36 addresses the education, training and effective use of all human resources for health for all, with a strong emphasis on the philosophy and practice of primary health care and on response to community needs.

Public health leadership and infrastructure   Target 34 addresses the need for health for all development to be guided and coordinated. This becomes increasingly important as the need for long-term strategies in health becomes clearer, as health care systems become more pluralistic in the funding and ownership of institutions and services, and as health for all principles are gradually seen as having wide application in practice. As strategies on lifestyles, the environment and health services mature, the accompanying investment choices become correspondingly more complex and difficult. This creates a greater need for institutions to have strong public health mandates that facilitate these choices and stimulate necessary action.

Partnerships for health for all   Community participation and intersectoral action are fundamental principles of health for all. Participation encompasses many activities, from those of local self-help groups to the advocacy role played by voluntary organizations at regional and national levels. Target 37 addresses the structures and organizational processes that might be adopted in and by countries to facilitate the forging of partnerships for health for all. The underlying motive is to provide groups and public, private and voluntary bodies with access to decision-making on health, and to give them the support they need to become effective partners.

Consensus on ethics   The growing range of medical treatment and technology, with significant and differing resource implications, raises an increasing number of ethical issues and challenges established value systems. The issues concern policy, the rights of individuals and groups, and the effects of specific health care interventions. Target 38 proposes a commitment to take ethical considerations fully into account in health policy and practice. This can be done by establishing mechanisms that facilitate open discussion and accountability to the public.

Target 32 – Health research and development

By the year 2000, health research should strengthen the acquisition and application of knowledge in support of health for all development in all Member States.

> *This target can be achieved if Member States:*
>
> - *formulate specific health research strategies based on the guidelines for health for all research developed by the European Advisory Committee on Health Research;*
>
> - *set priorities for the acquisition and application of knowledge in health promotion, disease prevention, environmental health, health care and health for all development;*
>
> - *involve researchers, care providers, managers and community groups in the development of research strategies and priorities;*
>
> - *strengthen communication and cooperation between the scientific community and decision-makers in the application of new knowledge to health for all development.*

Problem statement   The countries of the Region are in a singularly advantageous position for producing sound and relevant knowledge in the health, life and social sciences that can be used to support health for all in the Region and throughout the world. Research is supported by numerous organizations, governmental and nongovernmental, at national and international levels. A vast research potential is concentrated in universities and diverse public and private research institutions *(2)*.

The need for health research   The rapid development of new knowledge in the life sciences has dramatically affected our capacity to intervene in the natural processes of life and increasingly raises profound ethical questions. It also tends to blur the boundaries between basic and applied research. A number of recent developments in the European Region also highlight the gap between decision-making needs and available scientific knowledge. For example, the serious ecological problems affecting many countries and their people call for intensified multidisciplinary research to support action programmes. The AIDS pandemic is a complex problem requiring sustained research to develop effective prevention and treatment. The questions raised about the long-term effects of low-dose radiation in the aftermath of the Chernobyl disaster indicate that gaps in scientific knowledge may be costly in both economic and social terms. Cardiovascular disorders, cancer, mental illness and health-damaging behaviour are a continuing burden on the countries of the Region. This is a reminder of the need for a better understanding of the fundamental mechanisms of human biology and behaviour as a basis for prevention *(3)*.

The relationship between the rising costs of health care and equity, the further development of health care systems in the Region and, in particular, the major restructuring of health services in the countries in the central and eastern part of the Region, all emphasize that health research should have a much stronger role. Research that focuses on practical problems is particularly needed. It can draw on the insights and methods of different disciplines, including epidemiology, information science and evaluation, management sciences, health economics and organizational behaviour.

Resistance to health research   Despite the need, the impressive research potential in the Region has not so far been tapped to support major health goals and programmes. The development and implementation of policies on health for all research in countries will probably continue to encounter obstacles and constraints. Some of these can be removed or attenuated through better dialogue and cooperation. Others will require special efforts to change attitudes and behaviour and initiate institutional change.

Few countries in the Region have adopted explicit policies to carry out health research aimed at agreed targets and to make use of its problem-solving capacity. Many policy- and decision-makers do not sufficiently understand the role and potential of health research, particularly in relation to health for all development. Its role in the achievement of the regional targets is not readily perceived. Even in countries with long-standing traditions of high quality scientific research, policy-makers often tend to concentrate on the costs rather than the benefits of research. They also overlook the opportunities for achieving more effective and less costly solutions to health problems through relevant research. One inevitable result is a low level of funding for health research.

Resistance to evaluative research is a special problem. Once launched, a health care programme is difficult to change, because it usually involves a considerable investment of material and human resources, professional prestige and high expectations. Research for health for all tries to find out why systems or programmes succeed or fail. Some policy- and decision-makers and programme managers may well see this as a potential threat.

For their part, some scientists are reluctant to be involved in target-directed health research. They may also argue that any research policy infringes scientific and academic freedom. Researchers are typically independent-minded and few are ready to become involved in activities directly related to policy development. They fear that policy-makers and administrators will want instant results, while they are unwilling to commit themselves until their hypotheses and theories have been adequately tested.

Problems in research coordination and management   Insufficient communication and interaction takes place between existing research organizations and networks in the Region. One consequence of this is that certain types of study are seldom undertaken. These include longitudinal studies, studies of small area variation, and collaborative studies that are important in developing strategic knowledge. These are best carried out collaboratively by a number of often international research centres that share common objectives, methodology and research instruments.

The coordination of research within countries is also inadequate. It is often supervised by ministries responsible for science or education, which are not always aware of the value of health for all. In addition, the task of coordinating the work of different partners – universities, research councils, foundations, industry and independent research institutions – can be delicate and complex. A central objective of the various partners in research policy should be to achieve a proper balance between medical and public health research. Some countries have no central research policy bodies. In others, medical research councils tend to support basic and clinical, but not behavioural and public health research. The lack of adequate research funding inhibits the creation of a career structure in public health research, which is essential if high quality applicants are to be attracted into research training. In the vicious circle so created, research could not be carried out because of lack of trained personnel, even if adequate funding were to become available.

Ineffective research management is a major hindrance in the central and eastern part of the Region. The new governments have inherited an overcentralized, hierarchical and bureaucratic system of research planning and management. These countries have no tradition of schools of public health that combine education with research or with a service and consultancy function. Consequently, the link between advanced research and higher education is poor. Although the research in these countries has potential, its productivity and effectiveness are low, and hitherto researchers have had little motivation to be innovative. Many of these countries are trying to align their research management systems with the pattern of science management and funding that prevails in the rest of the Region. But this will only partially help promote and sustain research for health for all.

Suggested solutions   The main concern in society today is change. Research policies need to anticipate change and predict its consequences. They must also create timely solutions to new problems and adapt to new needs. Not all intellectually interesting research topics deserve support. Priority should be given to health for all research that is:

- scientifically sound, important and likely to be successfully performed;
- carried out on problems that have high human, social and economic cost, that are of epidemiological significance (such as avoidable

mortality, morbidity or disability) and that can easily be solved by using the results of research;
- relevant to the achievement of regional or country targets.

In 1988, the thirty-eighth session of the Regional Committee endorsed two documents, on research policies for health for all and on priority research for health for all *(4,5)*. Together, these documents continue to offer countries a framework in which to develop or update their health for all research policies and identify research priorities.

Identifying research needs   Issues for research should be identified in each of the clusters of targets supporting the regional health for all strategy. The precise assessment of priorities should emerge from discussions within countries between the research community and the health sector at various levels.

This debate will confirm the need for research to achieve better health (targets 1 – 12) in such areas as:

- barriers to equity and the sources of inequity; the measurement of inequities; the evaluation of policies designed to reduce inequities;
- the measurement of health status and quality of life; the identification of health needs; risk factors for disease; the impact on health of policies and activities in other sectors;
- the course and outcome of different illnesses and the effectiveness and efficiency of various forms of intervention.

Regarding lifestyles conducive to health (targets 13 – 17), research is required on:

- factors encouraging and discouraging different types of health behaviour; indicators of health-related behaviour; the meaning of health-damaging behaviour for the individual and its purpose for the individual and society;

— attitudes in the community towards health and health policies, and mechanisms for community involvement; social networks, formal and informal community structures and the distribution of power;
— the evaluation of intervention programmes.

Environmental health (targets 18 – 25) will require research on:

— specific environmental agents and their effects; risk assessment and management; integrated monitoring systems.

Appropriate care (targets 26 – 31) will require research on:

— the organization and management of care at different levels; the options determining a public/private mix of resources and provision of care; resource allocation models and the balance of resources between primary and other levels of care;
— the evaluation of the education and training of health care personnel, of health technology, and of health services performance; the quality of care, the acceptability of health services to patients and the public, and the relations between providers and patients;
— the mobilization of community participation, the role of lay care and self-help as such and in relationship to professional care; the financial and emotional costs of illness to families and patients.

Health for all development strategies (targets 32 – 37) will require research on:

— mechanisms for developing health policy; societal factors influencing the design and implementation of health policy, including motivation and incentive for policy change;
— the development of information systems including the definition of concepts and units of measurement, and the methods and scope of health reporting; the availability, reliability and interpretation of data; the development of better indicators for evaluating progress towards health for all;
— organization and decision-making in health for all development, especially at the community level, and their relation to intersectoral collaboration.

Target 38 on ethics and health will require research on:

— ethical issues and trends in health policies and actions and their consequences for the treatment of individuals;
— the ethics of research involving human subjects.

Promoting health for all research   The promotion of health for all research requires many partners. Ministries of health, education, research and science, as well as universities, medical and other research councils, private foundations, intergovernmental organizations and nongovernmental scientific societies all have a part to play. A health for all research policy will be successful only if the research community knows about it and accepts it. Several countries provide encouraging examples of successful national meetings arranged to discuss the implications of health for all for the research community. Scientific societies can play an important role in making regional and country health for all research policies known through their journals, conferences and meetings. Many international and national journals have reviewed the documents on the European health for all policy. The International Epidemiological Association, the Association of Medical Deans in Europe, the Association of Schools of Public Health in the European Region, the European Healthcare Management Association and several national scientific societies of health professionals have included sessions on research for health for all in their meetings *(6 – 8)*.

The research community needs incentives to carry out research in support of health for all. Some countries may consider establishing research councils and competitive grant application systems, while others may promote the idea of guided and targeted research. Structures should be established to promote closer cooperation between researchers and the managers of health and social welfare services. An essential requirement is that health authorities in each country publicly express their commitment to health for all research.

Resources and means to sustain health for all research   New forms of cooperation are needed to promote the multidisciplinary work between the sciences that is essential to research for health for all. Scientific institutions should be organized in a way that allows them to respond to society's basic health needs and to support its policies. For instance, all disciplines relevant to health should be represented in a country's medical research council, and universities should support people in different disciplines who wish to work together.

Universities are particularly important for the promotion and implementation of health for all research. They can:

– set up interdisciplinary research working groups;
– develop programmes to train personnel in new forms of research and in applying research findings in health care and health-related areas; and
– help individuals, other universities and related institutions, organizations and countries to exchange information, experience, research plans, programmes and findings.

Special research institutes, new professorships, peer review of research papers and better research training have often helped to promote new fields and attract talented young researchers. Training programmes need to be expanded and improved in several disciplines related to public health, such as: community and social medicine; social sciences related to health; epidemiology and statistics; systems analysis, health economics and operational research; and toxicology and environmental risk assessment. There is considerable scope for international collaboration on training. Health services research and epidemiology training courses would be particularly useful for the countries in the central and eastern part of the Region.

The allocation of adequate resources is the best incentive to research. Such an allocation should reflect the country's health research policies and health for all priorities. Training in research management will increase the effectiveness with which large, multidisciplinary projects are carried out.

Communication and coordination   Communication between researchers, health policy-makers and professionals is vital if each group is to have a better understanding of the others' needs. Opportunities for each to see the others at work, as well as special events to bring the groups together, can help improve communication. It may be possible to establish joint bodies to review the results of current research, to identify needs for new research and to establish scientific advisory posts for high-level decision-makers.

Finally, countries should consider how WHO, through its network of collaborating centres and its joint work with other international organizations and associations, can stimulate and assist the development of research policies and coordinate international cooperative ventures. The European Advisory Committee on Health Research is well placed to promote throughout the Region the ideas underlying research for health for all.

Target 33 – Health for all policy development

By the year 2000, all Member States should have developed, and be implementing, policies in line with the concepts and principles of the European health for all policy, balancing lifestyle, environment and health service concerns.

This target can be achieved if, after full consultation with the partners concerned:

- *health for all policies are adopted and continuously adapted at country, regional and local levels that are suited to the specific political and administrative structure of the country;*

- *specific targets are set for the achievement of health for all, reflecting the economic, social and cultural circumstances of the country concerned;*

- *those targets support greater equity in health, wider participation in decision-making, stronger emphasis on health promotion and disease prevention, effective intersectoral action, and reorientation of health services towards primary care (see Chapter 1);*

- *policies and targets are accompanied by specific strategies for their implementation, including legislation where appropriate;*

- *strong political commitment to such policies is affirmed at the highest level and reflected in legislation;*

- *Member States base their collaboration in international transactions, agreements and supranational policy-making on the principles of health for all.*

Problem statement   All Member States endorsed the principles of a common health policy when the regional strategy for attaining health for all was approved by the Regional Committee in 1980. Almost all countries have since begun to consider how to apply these principles in their own situation. A number have adapted their health policies and, where necessary, their legislation in accordance with health for all principles. Now is the time to assess this experience of health for all policy development and to identify desired future developments. When the targets were proposed in 1984, a widely perceived impression, especially in pluralist countries, was that many targets required central government direction and control. This impression has been modified to a considerable extent by the working group of pluralist countries, in cooperation with the WHO secretariat, which demonstrated that health for all policy development is not intrinsically centralist *(9)*. Many countries are now undergoing political change, involving either devolution or some significant degree of decentralization or regionalization. The health policy-making arena will be transformed in these countries. Policy-makers, whether reforming the health care system or contemplating other policies and actions to improve the population's health, can profit from the experience to date of the pluralist countries.

Country experience in health for all policy-making   Over half the countries in the Region have drawn up specific, countrywide policies and strategies that relate to the subject areas covered in the regional strategy. The policy documents that have been prepared have had varying purposes and political weight. Some make largely symbolic mention of health for all, while in others it is a constant reference point for policy development and resource allocation. Others see health for all as a framework for the integration of different issue-specific policies and as guidance for more local levels and for the private sector.

Some countries adopted the regional targets while others defined their own quantified country-specific targets. Some preferred non-quantified policy statements better suited to their political and cultural environment. Other countries that have not yet developed an explicit, comprehensive health for all policy have, even so, included in their periodic national health status reports a section on progress towards the regional targets.

A number of countries, as part of their overall efforts to implement health for all, are developing issue-specific policies in line with its principles. These policies focus on, for example, relevant research, food and nutrition, or the environment and health. In some countries, policies relating mainly or exclusively to health care have been developed, but not analogous policies on lifestyles and the environment. Conversely, in some places, policies have been developed for health promotion, although health services are not in line with health for all principles.

Operationally, it has often been difficult for national and subnational health for all policies to cover all the 38 targets at the same time *(10)*. Where attention at the country level has focused on a restricted number of issues, this has often been because of limited capacity and not necessarily the result of an explicit priority-setting and decision-making process. At the subnational level, economic constraints in practically all countries seem to have resulted in a more conscious effort to set explicit priorities, and there have been good examples of priorities set by defined criteria *(11)*. Even so, special attention needs to be given to improving equity between subnational levels.

In summary, many countries have still to produce a comprehensive set of policies covering all facets of the regional strategy (lifestyles, the environment and health care). In all cases, inequities in health, rapid developments in medical technology, and significant social and economic changes affect the burden of ill health and the need for care. They are creating serious ethical and other problems with which health policy must contend.

Policy process difficulties   More often than not, small groups of interested people have initiated the health for all policy formulation process, but they cannot sustain their enthusiastic commitment indefinitely when this is not their main responsibility. Further improvements in the process and mechanisms for policy formulation, implementation, monitoring and evaluation are needed throughout the Region.

Insufficient attention has been paid to the production, presentation and use of information for policy-making. Information must be presented in a format and manner appropriate to each target audience *(11)*. This is a crucial condition for wider participation in decision-making at an early stage of policy development, for the active involvement of stakeholders, particularly those in other sectors, and for the management of possible conflicts of interest. Short-term, incremental steps taken in health care reforms and development are not always checked for their consonance with long-term health goals. The responsibility for policy implementation may not be clearly designated, nor the necessary resources allocated.

Anticipating policy problems   The movement of people, goods and services across national borders is being encouraged in the part of the Region covered by the European Economic Area. The breaking down of barriers will, however, create new challenges for health policy. For example, the free movement of people may encourage more "medical tourism" (people travelling from one country to another for treatment). The free circulation of health professionals may add to the existing maldistribution of human resources in some countries. The free circulation of potentially health-damaging goods and services may help sustain unhealthy lifestyles.

The political and economic changes occurring throughout the Region mean that countries that had formulated health for all policy documents may need to revise them. In the central and eastern part of the Region, this will entail wide-ranging legislative changes, including changes in their constitutions, as the health sector joins the general move to a new economic and political system. These legislative changes will be of a scale that goes far beyond what is usual at any one time in a country and will take many years to complete, making heavy demands on legal, policy and economic expertise.

Suggested solutions   The regional health for all policy provides a comprehensive yet flexible framework, that can be adapted to suit different socioeconomic, political, cultural and administrative settings. It should therefore prove particularly suited to the central and eastern part of the Region where health policy changes form part of a radical review of all socioeconomic policy. When they adopted the regional strategy, all the Member States undertook to report on their progress to the Regional Office, thus also facilitating the exchange of experiences between countries *(3,12 – 14)*. This has begun to create a strong base of knowledge on how to apply health for all principles in different policy-making contexts. This foundation can now be built on in the new climate of more free and open reporting, particularly from the central and eastern part of the Region, and of greater receptiveness throughout the Region to fresh ideas.

Elements of good practice Countries' cumulative experience in health for all policy-making offers certain pointers to future good practice. An essential step is the process of formulation and periodic review of policies. These policies may be contained in one comprehensive policy statement or in a series. Policy statements emphasize political commitment to the health for all concept and principles, and provide the sense of strategic intent and the long-term framework within which operational targets and other short-term measures can be developed. They facilitate the overall coordination and integration of issue-specific policies and strategies, and focus attention on the intended outcomes of policy and action.

The financial constraints expected in the decade ahead indicate a pressing need to set explicit priorities. Some difficult choices will have to be made, guided by the fundamental health for all values and principles. While policies may not cover all the regional targets at once, a schedule can be set to cover various packages of targets, building up to a comprehensive health for all policy to cover all facets of the strategy.

In a number of countries, the preparation of health status reports has proved to be a valuable first step in policy formulation. Such information can sensitize all partners to health issues in a wide societal context, to the importance of the prerequisites for health, and to the existence of continuing inequities in health status and in access to health services. In some countries, such reports have been regularly produced and presented to parliament, which has been extremely effective in sensitizing the legislators to health policy. Public health research and action plans on specific issues, including health service reforms, can also be important entry points into the process of developing a comprehensive policy based on health for all.

Setting targets is one of the instruments for policy formulation and public health development. Targets should define the outcome to be achieved, be simple and easily understood, explain policy direction and emphasis, guide work and foster target setting at other levels in the country, and be based on scientific evidence rather than political expediency. Target setting is one of the ways to involve and influence partners, be they ministries at the national level or schools at the local level, and to create a common focus of interest and action (see also target 37). It is an instrument that can be used in a flexible and adaptable manner, is politically suited to the pluralistic societies of the Region, and enhances independent action and innovation among the many groups that work on projects.

Target setting and the development of indicators for monitoring should ensure that the initial policy formulation stage focuses on evaluation. The cyclical nature of policy development suggests that monitoring and evaluation can be assigned to a particular person or group. Where this responsibility has been given to a specific unit within a health administration, an active and vital focal point for health for all has been created. But steps must also be taken at political and managerial levels to ensure that it is the focal point and not the only point of activity. Policy development must be a shared responsibility among many interested partners.

Given the intersectoral character of much health policy, the ministry or other authority responsible for health must take the initiative in encouraging and supporting policy development in other sectors that is in line with health for all principles *(15)*.

Lessons from practical experience   Wide participation through a broad consultation process, with transparent mechanisms for feedback, can counter resistance and break down sectoral barriers. This involves conscious outreach to opinion-formers and decision-makers in other sectors, and patient negotiation with key ministries (particularly finance) to identify trade-offs between health and other objectives and to clarify the criteria for determining priorities. Reported examples of effective solutions include the following.

1.   The head of government chairs a health policy formulation committee, thus ensuring it has status and political significance and reflects the intersectoral nature of the process.

2.   Consultations are instituted without specifying the intended outcomes beforehand. They bring together participants from various interests and focus on alternative futures and scenarios rather than prepared draft policies and strategies. They consider the mutual interests of health and other sectors and the links between health, social, economic and other policies.

3.   Regional meetings are organized throughout the country to consider the opinions expressed by different interests and to reach conclusions that can build up into a national policy.

4.   In some countries with pluralistic systems, consensus meetings are convened of all the main partners in policy implementation (professional associations, nongovernmental organizations, insurance organizations and health service bodies).

5.   Policy statements at the national and subnational levels are used as a rallying point to mobilize nongovernmental organizations, professional associations, the academic and research communities, and individuals in key positions as opinion-formers, all of whom can influence decision-making.

6.   Local citizens' study groups are established and properly briefed, ensuring that their involvement begins with problem definition and follows through into implementation of solutions.

7.   Health for all policy documents are summarized to facilitate their discussion by the legislature. Popular versions are distributed to the general public at the same time. This achieves broad public participation in the policy debate and strong political affirmation of health for all policies at the highest level, which can be enacted in legislation.

Importance of local policy-making   In a number of countries, health for all policies developed at the regional and also municipal level (often in the context of a local Healthy Cities project) provide the most effective mechanisms for intersectoral action and wide participation in decision-making. These policies offer a powerful means of achieving both countrywide health objectives and those geared to specific regional conditions. The approaches adopted have frequently been innovative *(11)*. Through the exchange of experience with others and with support from the central or federal level, they have the potential for a significant synergistic effect. When decentralizing policy development, mechanisms must also be established to deal with issues of equity. The very focus on local policy and action will inevitably bring into sharp relief existing inequities in health and the plight of disadvantaged groups.

Policy implementation   As the experience in the Region shows, the setting of specific (and, when appropriate, quantitative) targets facilitates debate, the rallying of partners and the initiation of action. It also shows that at all levels, a clear strategy for the implementation of policy is necessary. Possible problems and conflicts of interest should be considered in the formulation phase, and responsibility and accountability designated clearly *(16)*. This can be achieved by direct discussion with the potential partners in implementation, through consensus meetings or other means.

When the magnitude of the change to a policy based on health for all is great, it requires time, patience and perseverance. Such a policy requires an approach that focuses in the first instance on outcomes and health, rather than on the provision of health services. This usually entails changes in attitudes and behaviour not only in the health care system, but in other sectors and in community groups and individuals. These changes are not always easily achieved, and when achieved not easily sustained. Decisions are constantly made – both nationally and internationally, inside and outside the health sector – that affect the health of the population. Continuous effort is essential to ensure that they respect health for all values.

Target 34 – Managing health for all development

By the year 2000, management structures and processes should exist in all Member States to inspire, guide and coordinate health development, in line with health for all principles.

This target can be achieved in all Member States if:

*   *responsive institutions are established with strong public mandates to act as public health advocates and to guide and coordinate health development at country, regional and local levels;*

*   *problem and priority definition is based on assessment of population health status, the prevalence of social and environmental risks, and the evaluation of health system performance;*

*   *processes are put in train to strengthen intersectoral commitment to greater investment in health and the attainment of priority targets;*

> • *a long-term perspective is adopted in target setting, strategic planning and evaluation, together with a readiness to respond to changing circumstances;*
> • *health system performance is evaluated in terms of achievement of improved health status, quality of life, public satisfaction, cost-effectiveness and health for all targets.*

Problem statement   A managerial infrastructure is required that will guide and support health development, implement health for all policies and sustain progress towards that goal. Management in many countries concentrates on health care, i.e. medical services, rather than on the overall health system or the set of actions needed to prevent and control disease, to promote health, to provide care and to support health development, regardless of where that action occurs in society. More attention should be given to managing the health system, identifying what health development steps are required and charting the most cost-effective path towards health for all.

Major health sector reforms are often aimed more at improving the management of hospitals than at the more complex tasks of improving the population's health. In several countries, the functions and status of public health departments and officials have declined, compared with those of their colleagues in clinical medicine who have easy access to decision-makers. Yet those working in medicine attribute less importance to population health than to the health of individual patients.

Until health for all policy becomes a central focus of management systems and priorities, the old, partial and segmented approaches will continue.

Creating a responsive management   Many countries had begun to promote participation in consensus development, planning and budgeting according to needs, and continuous adaptation to new circumstances by means of monitoring and reprogramming. Yet this process sometimes became stifled by creeping centralization, bureaucracy and rigidity. Countries are launching new initiatives throughout the Region to make public sector management systems more responsive to consumers and users of services *(17)*. They are investigating the role of the voluntary and private sectors with the aim of strengthening them. Interest has been renewed in decentralization, incentives, market-like mechanisms and relationships that free local management to experiment with new approaches. Such an approach requires simultaneous political and managerial effort to maintain the functioning of a public health infrastructure *(18)*.

Segmented managerial infrastructures and the lack of a system, or even an organizational focal point, with a comprehensive health for all perspective have made action outside the health services – such as advocacy directed at and partnership with industry – the exception rather than the rule. They have also created a culture of reactive management. The emphasis has been on the operational short term rather than the strategic long term, and on the resources and activities of institutions rather than the outcomes of actions. Problem- and cost-containment have been stressed instead of the cost-effectiveness of a whole set of initiatives in health protection and promotion, disease prevention, and environmental health improvement. Health action is rarely designed and implemented within an overall health for all framework.

Suggested solutions   It must be stressed at the outset that management, in the sense of coordination of health development, is not the same as operational control. Many private, voluntary and public bodies are engaged in health-related operations in different sectors and environments. Just as WHO has the constitutional mandate to coordinate and direct international health work so, within countries, a managerial structure and process are required to inspire and coordinate comprehensive health efforts.

Coordination, leadership and incentives   Various institutions and actors with leadership roles and public mandates have the task of inspiring and guiding health development in the implementation of health for all policies in countries. The backbone of a managerial structure at the national level is a ministry with responsibility for health. At the subnational level, the backbone is regional and/or local government departments of health or other public agencies. Examples also exist of interdepartmental bodies of various kinds, with important management or advisory functions, that operate at different levels and link different sectors of the economy. The Healthy Cities project, for instance, demonstrates the value of a local forum for the debate of health issues and for the integration of action by public health and other interests. Local public health offices with health protection and other community health functions can be valuable focal points for action.

Agencies and public officials with health mandates need persistently to advocate health for all values, principles and policies. Health will only attract and sustain political attention as a political issue when these values have been readily accepted by the leaders of the public, private and voluntary sectors.

Advocacy can also be delegated and institutionalized. It is not necessarily a public sector task. Indeed, advocacy has sometimes been converted into commercially successful advisory services to business.

While no single model for management and accountability can be used everywhere, extreme models of "central command" and "pure market" are equally unsuitable for health development. The central command model has been a failure in the central and eastern part of the Region and is unlikely to be replicated. Nowhere in the Region, on the other hand, does one find a pure market model untempered by any public intervention. Such an abrogation of all government responsibility towards the population would generate unacceptable social tensions and inequities *(19)*. Countries have to strive for a balance in health policy between guidance and autonomy, according to their legal, administrative, political and economic circumstances. Policy implementation has to be supported by regulatory, financial and other incentives, and at the same time has to allow autonomous action at various levels. If health for all advocacy has been effective, local action will be consonant with national health policy.

Managing for coherence and sustained action
A managerial infrastructure must be able to bring together and coordinate all functions, including the prevention and control of disease, health promotion, environmental health action, health care and health development support. The managerial aim in health for all is not a disaggregated, serial attack on targets one by one, but a cohesive programme of action in which identified problems and priorities attract rational responses. Each action programme should stimulate interest and sustain motivation

among public, private and voluntary sectors as appropriate, whether at the local, national or international levels.

Sound management practice, aligned to health for all principles, calls for problems, priorities and programmes to be defined on the basis of careful, well founded assessments of the current and anticipated health situation of the population. These assessments should cover health status, the prevalence of social and environmental health risk, and the efficiency, cost-effectiveness and equity of programmes at all levels of the health system, not just the health services. The implementation of the resulting action programmes must be suited to the local realities of political will, economic circumstances and the level of social development. This requires both a constant challenge to traditional health development approaches and the identification, testing and dissemination of effective innovations.

Investment in health pays   Generating intersectoral commitment to investing in health depends on structures and mechanisms that facilitate continuing dialogue and collaboration between health and other sectors, especially business and trade. The dialogue should focus on the ordinary settings of life (such as the workplace, the home and shopping areas) and emphasize the potential for collaboration on priority targets. The most powerful argument for action for and investment in health by other sectors is that of mutual benefit: health pays. Collaboration and investment in health are in the interest of all parties. For example, when the work environment becomes healthier, staff are more satisfied, labour turnover and absenteeism decrease, production uses technology less harmful to the environment, and a product or service may be

described as healthy or health-enhancing. A firm that demonstrates its sense of social responsibility may improve its standing in the community without losing its market share.

Partners not monoliths   The emphasis on generating intersectoral commitment fits well with the current trend towards decentralization, pluralism and accountability. It would be inappropriate and counterproductive to set up a monolithic infrastructure to support health for all. The managerial tasks involved require a range of knowledge, skills and information support and must respect the culture and values of all the people involved. It is good practice not to put all management functions into the same hands. Citizens' groups and the voluntary sector can develop and test many approaches before they become part of public practice. Business councils, trade unions, associations of health care providers and health insurance funds can be given authority to take up and deal with health issues in their own sectors. The aim in such cases is to promote a process of local action by the interested partners, following the principle of subsidiarity (according to which government steps in only if the process fails). Some countries have well developed systems for self-governance in the health services, involving physicians, insurers and health care institutions. Examples of self-governance outside the health services include different forms of risk community. These require businesses and organizations that create pollution and other health risks to assume joint liability for them. When their financial contribution is related to risk, they have an incentive to minimize that risk and use more appropriate technology.

The health for all concept and principles can rarely be integrated into economic and social development policies unless mutual interests are identified and respected. Nevertheless, some sectors are, on their own initiative, developing policies and strategies that benefit health. By publicly recognizing and commending these initiatives, the health sector can stimulate further action based on health for all principles. The health sector should also be willing to motivate other sectors to lead. It can achieve this by becoming more active in assisting other sectors and by recognizing explicitly the contribution to health of various public, private and voluntary bodies throughout society.

The need for a long-term perspective   Much action for health takes time to complete, especially projects such as safer roads, sewage disposal and other components of the physical infrastructure for public health. The long-term perspective also includes the periodic evaluation of projects in terms of better health, quality of life, services to vulnerable groups and better coverage and access. Similarly, creating conditions supportive of action for health, such as by building new social institutions, by seeking to move the values of various sectors closer to health for all, and by developing suitable professional training for managers, all takes time.

In managing action programmes, projected long-term outcomes and strategic thinking need to be reconciled with short-term objectives and day-to-day problem solving. Any initiative to reform health service structure or financing should, in particular, not proceed without regard for its impact on the population's health and its contribution to overall long-term health for all policies and aims.

A cadre of effective managers for health development   The long-term view requires proficient managers. They need not only to be strong in traditional functions such as personnel development, financial accounting and the timely discharge of business, but also to have a clear understanding of their role in health development. Such executives need to acquire health-specific management skills such as assessments of health status and quality of life, quality development and the assessment of health systems performance. They should be familiar with the economic evaluation of policy options, strategic resource allocation, and efficiency and effectiveness measures in the health sector. Their success in progressing towards the attainment of the health for all targets will continue to be evaluated by these criteria.

Target 35 – Health information support

By the year 2000, health information systems in all Member States should actively support the formulation, implementation, monitoring and evaluation of health for all policies.

This target can be achieved if there are information strategies in Member States that:

- *use appropriate indicators to measure progress towards targets for health policy outcome and programme performance;*

- *provide for intelligence systems to forecast future problems and needs;*

- *provide for minimum data sets based on internationally agreed standards, including data for measuring achievement of regional health for all targets;*

- *facilitate information exchange with other sectors and provide politicians, managers, interested groups and the public with relevant information;*

- *are based on appropriate use of information technology.*

Problem statement   Since the adoption of the health for all strategy, the countries of the Region have become more aware of the need for adequate information for policy formulation, implementation and monitoring. The adoption of the regional targets and indicators resulted in the establishment of a regular monitoring and evaluation process. The experience of three such exercises has helped countries to see their information needs more clearly *(3,12 – 14)*.

Significant technological progress has occurred in publishing, personal computers and telecommunications. For example, laser disc databases, electronic publishing and artificial intelligence facilitate the storage, processing and transfer of information. Some progress has also been made in the standardization of data processing and communication procedures to overcome technological incompatibilities between different equipment and software.

Lack of progress in developing health information systems   Despite the progress made in technology, and the efforts of some countries to develop national health information policies, information support in a number of countries is still far from satisfactory: it is not geared towards supporting health policy and action. In these countries, the collection, analysis and publication of data reflect the priorities of the past, rather than present and future needs. Many health information systems require further development, particularly in the central and eastern and some of the southern part of the Region.

Nearly all health systems suffer from information overload, in that few of the data collected and generated can be processed, transformed into information and used. There is an avalanche of data but much of it is of limited use for health development. Information overload is an unnecessary burden on time and resources.

Information for a purpose   Too little emphasis is placed on the transformation of data into information, knowledge and intelligence, and on effective presentation and feedback to the users who are supposed to take action. Policy- and decision-makers may be said to be "drowning in data" and, at the same time, to be starved of relevant infor-mation *(20)*. There are a number of explanations. Different components of health information sys-tems, such as registers, surveys, health services information and scientific information, have de-veloped separately. They are uncoordinated and incompatible. The needs of small areas and local level management are often considered secondary to central level reporting requirements.

Information in the health services is often geared only to the allocation of resources and the control of spending, not to the need to evaluate services and patient outcomes. Population-based data – on morbidity, disability, the use of services, lifestyles and positive health – have not received the atten-tion their importance warrants. All these factors point to the need for research and development in a number of areas, such as information on health status and the quality of life. Better indicators should be developed for wellbeing and perceived health status, morbidity, disability, the control and use of various resources, and the quality and acces-sibility of services.

Networks for the exchange and dissemination of health documentation, which are important for ef-fective information support, do not always function. Some countries, particularly those in the central and eastern part of the Region, still lack reliable, rel-evant, up-to-date information for policy and other purposes. They must now build up the necessary capacity both to generate and to use information.

Suggested solutions   The shift towards a more integrated Europe will create greater oppor-tunities for cooperation and information exchange, both within the European Community and in the Region as a whole.

Cooperating for information support   Through-out the regional strategy and each of its 38 targets, information is identified as a key resource for success. The fortieth session of the Regional Committee for Europe in 1990, in resolution EUR/RC40/R6, adopted a European health for all infor-mation strategy *(21)* calling for integrated in-formation support in Member States and the Re-gional Office. Such a strategy should clearly state how the information will be used for each of the major components of health for all. It should mobi-lize the resources to be devoted to information support, specify the structure and management of the information system and determine the mech-anisms for data collection, analysis, quality, com-munication, access, retrieval and reporting. It should also determine the most appropriate forms of communication and presentation and include an evaluation of the quality, cost-effectiveness and impact of health decisions and actions.

An advisory body, with representatives from all concerned parties, can establish effective liaison between authorities and facilitate the formulation and implementation of the strategy. The strategy should cover the collection, processing and deliv-ery of relevant information to all potential partners in health development. Wherever feasible, quanti-fiable targets for health action and indicators to measure progress should be adopted. They give the reference framework for priority-setting and any necessary reorientation of the health system. They may also enable comparisons to be made between populations, geographical areas and agencies re-garding levels of health and the performance of the health system.

The scope of information required   Information should also be available on the social and physical environment relevant to health. A multisource health intelligence system encompassing both hard and soft types of information should be developed for use in forecasting or anticipating future conditions, problems and needs. Population survey information is essential to monitor health attitudes and behaviour and to measure the level of satisfaction with services. This information can be incorporated into health reports at all levels. More emphasis could also be given to population-based registers for chronic diseases such as cancer, cardiovascular diseases and mental disorders, which must safeguard the anonymity of individual patients.

The formulation of programmes and the evaluation of performance require hazards and risks (particularly in the living and working environments) to be linked to health. Costs and activities have to be related to outcome, in terms of improvements in protection achieved and in the health, attitudes and behaviour of the population. Data must often be linked to become meaningful information. For example, the quality and appropriateness of care in the health services can only be assessed by focusing on a total episode. Looking at the individual activities or technical components is insufficient. Sometimes, existing data could be better used in meta-analysis: by judiciously aggregating and re-analysing to generate further insights. But, equally important, whatever the preceding analysis, information in support of decision-making has to be presented effectively to the intended audience.

Building the information system   Perhaps the most important element of an information service is the appropriate communication and use of the information. Communication must be improved between originators, user groups and other interested parties *(22)*. A permanent focal point or unit can usefully be

established to act as a reference centre for potential users and providers of information. Information should be timely, purposeful and easily accessible. Building and using networks of institutions, agencies and lay informants optimizes the use of existing databases and documentation. At the same time, confidentiality must be protected and due attention paid to copyright and data ownership. A bottom-up approach is preferable. This involves local users in designing the system and in determining what data are to be collected and processed for decision-making and other purposes. If the people collecting the source data do not believe it is useful, they will have no real commitment to reliable, accurate and timely reporting.

When information systems are reviewed, adjusted or built, minimum data sets need to be defined for each area of health action. Countries and intergovernmental organizations need to cooperate among themselves to standardize definitions and coordinate data handling. It would also be valuable if they organized international consultations to develop common methods and to conduct health interview surveys, such as those already carried out by WHO in cooperation with the Netherlands Central Bureau of Statistics *(23)*. The monitoring and evaluation of progress towards health for all in the Region will continue to contribute significantly to this process of alignment, as will the information and telematics research activities of the European Community.

The role of the Regional Office   National and local agencies and institutions with health responsibilities may wish to consider how they can benefit from the activities and products of the Regional Office and its mandate as a European health information centre. A number of databases are being further developed and strengthened. Information packages are compiled and prepared on, for example, health promotion programmes, diabetes management and food safety. In future this work will also include knowledge development and forecasting.

The network of specialized information centres in selected programme areas should be expanded and more effectively used, and the exchange and dissemination of health information in the Region should be improved through national documentation centres. Electronic networking, as demonstrated by the Regional Office's WHONET, is a promising approach to increasing services, including database access, electronic mail, and bulletin board services.

Target 36 – Developing human resources for health

By the year 2000, education and training of health and other personnel in all Member States should actively contribute to the achievement of health for all.

This target can be achieved if, in the Member States:

- *basic and continuing education programmes for health personnel emphasize the principles and strategies of health for all and their application in practice;*

- *the objectives and values of health for all are communicated to other sectors relevant to health, for incorporation in their education programmes and their practice;*

- *basic and continuing education programmes place special emphasis on leadership development, encouraging participants to become health for all advocates.*

Problem statement   In many countries of the Region, human resource development does not fully reflect the needs of the community. There are surpluses and shortages of people of different professions and disciplines in different geographical areas.

Need rarely determines the number of personnel entering the training and health care delivery systems. In some cases, the number of doctors is increasing at such a pace that measures have already been taken to reduce future output from medical schools. Most countries in the Region now have over 200 doctors and 400 nurses per 100 000 inhabitants, but the ratio of doctors to nurses differs between countries. Even so, there can be gross geographical maldistribution. Doctors tend to congregate in economically prosperous areas in cities and the numbers training for specialist and primary care practice is unbalanced *(24)*.

Countries also differ widely in the availability of nurses, midwives, pharmacists and other health professionals. The number of nurses, for example, ranges from around 200 up to nearly 900 per 100 000 population. Some countries are seeing a faster increase in auxiliaries than in qualified nurses. It is increasingly difficult to recruit and retain nursing and other staff in caring roles, for various reasons: demographic trends, better financial and other rewards in other jobs, work-related stress and, not least, the ill-defined roles and functions in nursing. Some studies on the use of qualified nurses have suggested that no more than one fifth of their activity can be classified as nursing *(3)*.

Present practice in education and training A largely unchallenged belief exists that health care workers who are trained to some maximum level of scientific knowledge and technical skill will give a uniformly high quality service to the population. Generally speaking and until quite recently, little thought has been given to introducing a health for all perspective into the training of health workers or of their teachers *(25)*. Little interest has been shown in training them in aspects of public health either, or in emphasizing health professionals' leadership and management roles. Hospital-based medical education has dominated thinking on human resource development, reflecting the dominance of the medical specialist's perception of health problems and their technical management. Traditional institutions have given their students a knowledge base predominantly drawn from the biological and medical sciences, often with inadequate attention to the social and behavioural sciences and their relevance to health.

Both present teaching methods and the content of training can pose problems. Inadequacies can be quite fundamental, such as when training programmes fail to introduce students to the realities of people's needs and interests, and fail to integrate new knowledge and approaches from fields other than the biomedical.

Cooperation between the health care system and the institutions that train health professionals has often been inadequate. Fundamental expectations and attitudes among educators and practitioners alike have not been suited to the challenge of reorientation towards health for all values and objectives contained in Regional Committee resolution EUR/RC37/R7 on health personnel development. Health for all requires long-term development for the benefit of the whole population. It involves large numbers of public and private organizations, and covers a wide range of issues. Most health workers have, by training and temperament, narrower and more immediate goals in the care and cure of individuals.

The overall result of existing training policies and methods has been an overemphasis on producing specialists with very specific skills and competences, rather than generalists with broad vision who are adaptable and capable of integrating their own work with that of others, both within and outside the health sector.

Lack of contact with other sectors Little is known in the health sector about the current status of education on health and health-related matters in the curricula of other professionals. Given the prevailing lack of contact between educators of health professionals and other faculties in higher education, however, the curriculum content and learning materials are unlikely to inform these professionals about the impact of their work on health, or about the health for all strategy. Much closer cooperation is needed between the bodies responsible for policy-making and education in the health sector and their counterparts in other sectors. Since most training courses are already heavily burdened and there is little chance of lengthening courses, innovative ways will need to be developed to involve the trainees of other professions in the discussion of health for all principles and policies.

Suggested solutions   Every country needs a clear strategy for human resource development. It should take account of the country's particular socioeconomic conditions, but also reflect health for all values and goals *(26,27)*. To be effective, it will need to be developed in a coordinated way that is respected by all interests, that gives them a forum in which to negotiate and agree on the means of implementation, and that avoids associated problems such as oversupply, overspecialization and the inefficient use of personnel. The type of machinery adopted will depend on country circumstances, such as the distribution of responsibility within the health care system.

The core of such a strategy would be to ensure coordinated programmes for the training of health care personnel, based on scenarios or other reasoned projections of both health needs and labour market conditions.

The labour market   Planning and projecting human resource needs and availability is becoming both more difficult and more important. Predictions have to take into account the free movement of labour, particularly between countries in the European Economic Area, the international mutual recognition of professional qualifications, and the

possibility of substituting different categories of professional worker. It will be crucial to identify which groups of workers are ready to travel, from where and to where. The situation may be further complicated by countries with labour shortages offering attractive training and other opportunities to workers in countries with labour surpluses. Such developments should be pursued in a spirit of equity and international cooperation, avoiding the risk of one country feeling that its labour is being poached by another more advantaged country.

A training philosophy   Training, particularly the basic training of groups such as family doctors and community nurses, must be based on an understanding of and respect for the role and abilities of other health workers and their mutual dependence in teamwork. They should also learn to deal with the known and anticipated health problems of the population. If they are to contribute to health for all goals they must not only acquire professional and technical excellence but also:

– understand and accept health for all values and objectives as a framework for practical action that can be of continuing help in their daily work;

– acquire a foundation of integrated multidisciplinary knowledge and skills that go beyond the biological sciences to encompass behavioural, anthropological, social, economic and other fields as these relate to disease prevention, appropriate care and health protection and promotion (for example, the study of drug abuse integrates aspects of internal and forensic medicine, pharmacology, psychology, sociology and criminology);

– acquire leadership and teamwork skills that enable them to advise and collaborate with various authorities, community organizations and others in the development of health policies and campaigns;

— acquire communication and other skills for direct action with individuals or in the community in pursuit of health for all objectives; and

— develop the means of evaluating their own practice in terms of meeting the health needs of the community *(28)*.

Because education should be lifelong, continuing education underpinned by a mix of incentives and mandatory requirements must be a main thrust of a human resource strategy. Continuing education for family doctors and others should encompass health for all principles. It should also focus on changing health needs and policies and the appropriate application of new knowledge and technology. Most of the health professionals who will be working in the year 2000 are studying now or have already completed their studies. Given the scale of effort required, much continuing education must be based on self-learning, supplemented by some face-to-face contact with trainers.

A code of practice   In many countries professional training, especially continuing education for medical practitioners and other health professionals, has enjoyed financial and other support from commercial enterprises that sell their products and services to the health sector. The relationships so established and the help given have normally been marked by ethical conduct on all sides. They are nevertheless inherently delicate relationships, with a clear risk of conflict of interest. Countries should consider promoting a code of practice for support to educational and other forms of information disseminated to health professionals. The objective of a code of practice, while recognizing the valuable support

given, would be to ensure that trainers and training schemes remain independent of all forms of undue or improper external influence.

Ways and means in learning   Learning how to learn is important. Learning is always most effective and acceptable if it is active rather than passive, if it is perceived by the student to be relevant, and if it includes feedback on performance. Learning strategies that place the student in a practice setting and concentrate on problem identification and management satisfy these criteria. This points to the need for greater use of community settings in training and a shared commitment by the health care and other social service agencies, the professions and the training institutions. The evaluation of training programmes will need to focus on outcomes such as acquired skills and competences. This thereby ensures the trainees' learning matches the health needs of the community *(29)*.

If groups of students who are training for different professions share some learning activities, they have the opportunity to understand and appreciate each other's skills and improve their teamwork. For example, if the area of concern is care of the elderly, it makes sense that general practitioners, geriatricians, nurses, physiotherapists, psychologists and social workers all learn together *(30)*.

An international movement for change   In recent years, important initiatives have supported professional training based on health for all values and objectives. The favourable momentum needs to be sustained.

The Edinburgh Declaration of the World Conference on Medical Education, in 1988, pledged a "programme to alter the character of medical education so that it truly meets the defined needs of the society" *(31)*. The Region's ministers of health and of education issued the Lisbon initiative the same year, proposing that a country's medical education policy should reflect the regional health for all strategy; that educational programmes in individual universities and medical schools should reflect countries' health for all policies; that continuing education should become an essential feature of medical education; and that all phases of medical education should take place in appropriate settings that reflect all aspects of health and the health services *(32)*.

The Vienna Declaration on Nursing in Support of the European Targets for Health for All, made at the European Conference on Nursing in 1988, stated that:

> Nursing can best fulfil its potential in primary health care when nursing education provides a sound foundation for nursing practice, especially work in the community, and when nurses take account of the social aspects of health needs and have a broader understanding of health development *(33)*.

In partnership with WHO, the Association of Schools of Public Health in the European Region is producing curricula and learning materials for use in public health training based on health for all. The aim is to develop postgraduate vocational studies in a multidisciplinary field which encompass disease prevention, health protection and promotion programmes for populations, and the organization of cost-effective health services of high quality, with a particular stress on leadership, policy-making and management skills.

Making partners through training   Health for all also presents a challenge to professionals in other sectors. As partners in intersectoral collaboration, they must take full account of the impact of their activities on health and seek to attain their own goals in ways that will also protect and promote health. In view of the relative lack of effective links with workers in other sectors in the past, stress should be laid on developing the strategy to make fruitful contacts. While the definition of sectors varies between countries, a useful first step is to draw up an inventory of present and potential partners for health for all. The analysis should include the determination of which sectors would be likely to have the most impact on health, where key partners are easiest to identify, and where an approach is likely to be sympathetically received.

One way to generate interest in health for all values and objectives, and to secure their place in education and training programmes in other sectors, is to give visibility to an issue widely felt to be a matter of urgency. Training modules can then be developed that prompt these professionals to see the relevance of health for all approaches, particularly intersectoral partnerships and joint decision-making, and that stimulate them to acquire appropriate skills. The following are some examples of what this may imply for different professions and sectors.

Police officers and other law enforcement personnel should have an understanding of the psychosocial factors underlying social problems such as drug abuse. This will help them cooperate sympathetically with self-help groups, the community, and the health and social sectors.

When designing homes or planning neighbourhoods, architects should take account not only of their effect on general wellbeing, but also of the need to improve accident prevention, social contact and other health-promoting activities. Accident prevention can often be enhanced through relatively simple measures such as better lighting or the use of non-slip surfaces. The provision of ramps and handholds could also encourage elderly people to maintain their contacts and participate in social life.

Teacher training should include pedagogic techniques that help children develop the ability to make sound decisions and choose healthy lifestyles. Teachers themselves should understand the crucial influence of their own behaviour and of the school environment on their pupils.

The training of economists should give more emphasis to the cost to society of ill health, disability and premature death, and should include the application of cost-benefit and cost-effectiveness analysis to health matters.

Designers and civil engineers should be aware of the safety aspects of consumer goods and road design. Bioengineers should learn about the physical and psychological impact of technical devices used in health care. All of them should be aware of the less obvious effects of technology on lifestyles and health.

The potential of the media's role   With the removal of communication barriers in the Region, the role of the press, radio and television has acquired great importance. This is a field where media professionals in western Europe need to share their best practice and standards with their colleagues in the central and eastern part of the Region. Training events or briefings could usefully be organized to inform people in the media about the values and objectives of health for all. They could assess for themselves its rich potential in news, public information and education. Journalists and others, once aware of the principles and goals of health for all, can ensure that the mass media play an active role in giving effect to health for all strategies. Actors and other public entertainers who also have great influence on the general public should equally be approached and briefed when opportunities arise. Many may well then feel motivated to set a positive example by their own health behaviour and to refuse publicity, sponsorship offers and other assignments that promote or glamorize unhealthy habits such as smoking or excessive drinking.

Collaboration, participation, education   Managers and other leaders in the health sector increasingly appreciate that collaboration, like participation in all its forms, is educational and treat it as such. It generates understanding and helps build and sustain consensus on short- and long-term objectives. It should facilitate the elaboration of strategies that are both technically feasible and acceptable to the population. It can promote a sense of ownership, motivation and responsibility for the development of health for all programmes among a wide range of professional groups, policy sectors and individuals.

Education and learning about health for all can occur in many settings in different formats. In its broadest form it reaches all groups, makes health everybody's business, and stimulates them to action.

Target 37 – Partners for health

By the year 2000, in all Member States, a wide range of organizations and groups throughout the public, private and voluntary sectors should be actively contributing to the achievement of health for all.

This target can be achieved if broadly based active participation in health for all development is encouraged through structures and processes at the international, country, regional and local levels. This will require the involvement of a broad range of partners such as intergovernmental organizations, government departments, regional agencies, municipal authorities, professional organizations, industry and labour, and community groups. Partners will be gained through structures and processes that:

- *facilitate networking and communication between potential partners;*

- *provide access to priority-setting, planning, decision-making and implementation;*

- *place appropriate emphasis on decentralizing decision-making;*

- *widely disseminate information on health issues;*

- *provide support for the work of community groups;*

- *provide incentives that facilitate intersectoral action;*

- *strengthen international solidarity for European health for all development by using existing and emerging European structures for intergovernmental cooperation and action.*

Problem statement   An effective strategy of health development is based on a sound, comprehensive policy. Consistent with health for all principles, this policy must be supported by purposeful research and reliable, relevant information, and carried out by personnel who are properly trained and motivated by a service ethic that is inspired by health for all values. They must implement the strategy in a working environment that sensitively combines public, private and voluntary structures.

In all these facets of health development, the path to success lies in building partnerships.

Partnerships as a prerequisite   The implementation of the health for all policy relies heavily on the active commitment of many interests outside the health sector. The prerequisites for health include the provision of safe water and food, the design of safe homes and neighbourhoods, and the education of children to enable them to make wise choices about lifestyles. Specific health objectives, such as the reduction of alcohol consumption and of the prevalence of smoking, and greater social equity in the distribution of resources for health, can only be achieved if many sectors are involved.

Health for all is, as a matter of principle, a movement for people. They have the right to equal opportunity in health, the right to health care, the right to be informed, and the right to be involved as partners in decision-making and action affecting their health. Partnership for health means the encouragement of intersectoral collaboration and multisectoral action and the promotion of community participation. These have been regarded as fundamental to health for all, but none was taken up in practice as extensively as expected once the regional health for all strategy was adopted. Thus, this target addresses the issue by focusing on the need for fresh momentum in forging partnerships.

Many nongovernmental organizations, including self-help groups, and nearly all associations of health professionals have embraced health for all, and politicians in many municipalities have supported it. Nevertheless, few decision-makers in other sectors have been swayed to the point of shifting resources to meet or at least not to jeopardize health objectives. Much better communication and exchange of information is needed about positive experiences of joint action for health and of mechanisms for effective participation, which could have a multiplier effect in building true working partnerships.

Barriers to partnership   A number of barriers to partnership persist and there are several possible causes of failure. In any particular case, the specific cause must be identified if an appropriate solution

is to be found. In many cases, the mutual benefits to be obtained from commitment to health for all have not yet been presented in a sufficiently convincing way to all the main potential partners. Sometimes, the health policies of authorities at different levels are not sufficiently explicit or persuasive in arguing that health is the business of all sectors, not just the health sector. People working in sectors outside health, the mass media and the general public, often do not understand the concepts and principles of health for all, the specific problems to be addressed, the objectives being pursued and the means available to accomplish them, or the positive effect their cooperation would achieve.

The traditional arrangements for developing health policy and providing health care have often actively discouraged partnerships for health. Policy-making has been seen not as a cooperative task but as a technical task, the proper approach to which depended on specialist medical expertise and advice. Health care systems have often been noted for their tendency to exclude nonprofessional voices and to establish a social distance between professionals and the public. As a result of the closed organization and professionalization of health care, health workers themselves have failed to recognize opportunities to make partners and facilitate intersectoral investment in health.

The failure to find a common language to explain health issues to different groups is a serious problem. In many cases, the steps needed to facilitate communication between sectors and with the community and to develop a common knowledge base have not been deliberately examined. While human rights, including the protection of a patient's privacy, are inviolable, the principle of confidentiality has sometimes been used as a pretext to resist reasonable requests for information.

Partnership as an international challenge Beyond the arena of health care services, there is a further challenge to cement partnerships internationally in the policy areas of environmental health and the promotion of healthy patterns of living. Success in attacking major problems in both areas will depend on international solidarity. Chernobyl and other environmental disasters have made that crystal clear. In the lifestyles area, attention must focus on the consequences of the liberalization of the mass media and particularly the internationalization of television through satellite and cable. This means that both intended and incidental messages can instantly reach a growing audience Region-wide. These messages may be conveyed through both advertising and the role model images of popular figures in television films and entertainment programmes. Their behaviour may be health-promoting or -damaging. The poor environmental health record and the limited attention given to health promotion policies in the central and eastern part of the Region mean that a special international effort will be needed to support those countries. Overall, there are positive signs of international solidarity, but it is still too fragmented and uncoordinated to be as effective as it needs to be.

Encountering resistance At all levels, attempts to increase participation and develop partnerships for health have occasionally encountered resistance from politicians, bureaucrats and professional groups. They have justified their resistance by stating that existing mandates, legislation and systems of decision-making are functioning adequately, or that the new arrangements would be too slow and complex and the additional partners would not have the requisite technical competence and experience to make good decisions. More often

than not, the underlying reason has been that any moves to share decision-making challenge the existing distribution of power.

Suggested solutions The purpose of building partnerships and networks for health is to improve communications and ensure action outside the health sector. This networking may be accomplished in many ways.

Countries have found it constructive to facilitate participation through various political, public, private and voluntary bodies. Influential groups such as parliamentarians are showing an interest in health for all. They have strong potential as leaders of public opinion, and can be encouraged to advocate health for all, both in national and international parliaments and at home in their local constituencies. In countries with pluralistic health systems, the insurance organizations have been brought into the discussion and, in some countries, the trade unions are taking an interest. Religious organizations have traditionally played a strong role in the health care sector in many countries and can be expected to embrace a policy that emphasizes issues of equity, participation and involvement. It would be idealistic, however, to expect that participation and intersectoral action could be secured through the force of moral or ethical argument alone. Realistically, more attention must be given to uncovering and emphasizing the mutual benefits and particular advantages for each sector.

Examples have been reported of successful cooperation between government departments at the country, regional and local levels in encouraging the production of healthy food products, reducing environmental pollution, and coordinating health and social services. More recently, there has been a move to involve manufacturing and service industries in action for health. In some countries, butchers and supermarkets have begun to offer healthier food products, chefs have participated in training courses on healthy cooking, and some hotels and restaurants now prepare health dishes on a regular basis. Businesses are also workplaces, and an increasing number treat the solution of health problems as an investment in the health of the workers and the health of the business *(34)*.

Sustaining partnerships   Sharing information on health issues and establishing regular formal and informal communication is necessary to sustain partnerships. Communication grows out of working with partners to develop a common language and knowledge base and accepting the contributions of others drawn from their own knowledge and experience. In some places, adult education centres and courses have been used to involve people in the discussion of health for all. Local health facilities can be used as meeting places for interested individuals and groups. Many youth organizations have national and international networks that can be mobilized.

A crucial role for the media   A sustained effort is needed to mobilize all the resources of television and other modern means of communication to present the health for all concept and principles and the arguments for intersectoral action and community involvement. The potential of the media and their role in public education have not yet been properly tapped, but the possibilities are clear *(35)*. People in the media have much better communication skills than most health workers. By creating visibility for health issues, they can help sustain the political will to attain health for all objectives.

They can raise public awareness and explain and clarify options for action. Through audience participation and public access programmes, television in particular can feed public reactions back to policy-makers. People in the media aim to gain and retain the interest and sympathies of their audience. This need not conflict with the objectives of health policy-makers: they too have first to gain the public's attention if they are to inform, educate and persuade. In all circumstances, the way in which information is presented can be decisive. Information can be tailored to the needs of different target groups in the population and generate positive responses.

Implications of a partnership strategy   The partnership strategy will have different implications for the lifestyles, environment and health services targets because different partners will be identified, each with distinctive contributions to make. In each area, the strategy will need to identify which organizational structures and institutions can best support participation. Resources will have to be made available to make participation as attractive as possible. Winning partners for health requires the health sector to take conscious action to remove barriers and create arrangements that facilitate cooperation based on shared decision-making. In several countries, this will also mean strengthening the organizational and managerial capacity of public health departments and the strategic planning and evaluation function in the health sector.

One of the basic principles of networks and partnerships is that people have the right to be involved and informed. They ultimately decide on the value of health in their lives. Although the economic, social, cultural and physical environment may severely restrict their real options, people are partners in the health for all movement and they share responsibilities. They should be able to play an active role in seizing available opportunities to develop and maintain their health potential. With the right to be informed, they should be able to obtain information, to draw conclusions from it and to use it to exercise their influence.

People have a well established means of public participation in many countries: through self-help groups and voluntary organizations. These often operate on an informal basis with limited financial resources, depending on the time and energy of their membership (36). If such groups are to be effective participants, they require support in the form of information, technical assistance, network communication and financial aid. For example, in the area of health education, some national coordinating bodies offer research and training and lobby on behalf of a variety of voluntary organizations.

Successful partnerships at the local level   Where participation and partnership strategies have been adopted, the motivation in part has been to make health systems more responsive to local needs, to allow individuals and groups to set their own priorities, and to enlist the knowledge and resources of the community. Participation is most successful at the most local level. In some respects, the issues may be less complex than at the national level and can be clearly understood. Participation tends to operate more effectively in decentralized settings, where the people who make decisions are closer to the community and more sensitive to its needs. Local politicians and professionals are ready to respond to local groups concerned with a neighbourhood health problem. In several countries, the trend is towards allowing communities and neighbourhoods to decide

what they need from the health and social services, and to carry out plans through recognized committee structures. The Healthy Cities project (37,38) provides a positive example of cooperation between city departments steered by intersectoral committees of politicians and senior officials. An appropriate balance must be struck, however, between the two needs for central coordination and for decentralized participation.

The potential of international partnerships   At the international level, health has been moving to the forefront of the policy arena, stimulated by the common health policy for Europe. WHO's experience has shown the relevance, for health development in the Region, of making formal links with a number of nongovernmental organizations, such as through the European Forum of Medical Associations and WHO and the European Forum of Pharmaceutical Associations and WHO. Other important partnerships have been forged with the International Council of Nurses, the Association of Schools of Public Health in the European Region, the Association of Medical Deans in Europe and the International Diabetes Federation (European Region). Examples of WHO partnerships also include the networks of healthy cities, health-promoting companies, health-promoting schools and health-promoting hospitals.

Existing and emerging European integrational organizations will be striving to advance the wellbeing of all citizens in the Region through a process of consensus similar to that achieved by Member States in the Regional Committee. Popular pressure on international bodies is likely to extend beyond the established issues of disease prevention, drug abuse and environmental health and into demands for action to improve the quality of life.

All the political bodies pursuing Region-wide economic and social goals should therefore become potential partners in health for all. The Regional Committee and the Member States are pursuing a strategy of rapprochement in their policies and programmes with such organizations.

Target 38 – Health and ethics

By the year 2000, all Member States should have mechanisms in place to strengthen ethical considerations in decisions relating to the health of individuals, groups and populations.

The particular approaches adopted should be in accordance with the social and cultural characteristics of each country, and include:

- *the education and training of health professionals in ethics;*

- *measures to increase knowledge of ethical considerations among the public, politicians and other decision-makers;*

- *an ethical code of practice for health professionals, including the relationship between health care providers and patients;*

- *the strengthening of ethics bodies and other mechanisms at the appropriate levels and in relevant sectors that:*

  - *encourage widespread discussion of the interests of individual people, groups in the community, and the public at large;*

  - *specify and assess the ethical aspects of health policy, health care practice and health research and provide advice on them;*

  - *are free to speak independently from government, industry and professional or other particular interests, expressing their opinion on issues of health and ethics falling within their mandate;*

  - *facilitate open discussion and accountability to the public;*

  - *take full account of the health-related ethical principles contained in the Universal Declaration of Human Rights, the United Nations convention on human rights, the working decisions of the United Nations Commission on Human Rights and the recommendations of the Council of Europe.*

Problem statement   There has been an explosion of knowledge and technology in medical care. Some treatment and care can greatly increase life expectancy and the quality of life. Yet people have begun to ask whether medical action should have limits. At the same time, people have increasingly come to expect that medical technology will find a solution for every problem, including those that are social rather than medical. This has had a distorting effect: knowledge and technology have tended to be used only for closely defined, individual goals. For example, massive efforts are made to save the lives of premature infants while preventive primary care, which would address the quality of antenatal care and the living conditions of the mother, is ignored. This is basically an ethical issue.

In today's climate, ethical questions have to do not only with who shall have access to care and particular treatment and who, as a consequence, shall be denied such care. Such questions also increasingly apply to who shall have the opportunity to choose healthy lifestyles and who shall have access to healthy environments. Health for all presupposes that people should have maximum access and opportunity, at least as far as available resources allow. Its basic principle of equity is a reflection of a profound concern with ethics.

Who decides?   Ultimately, the question is who decides what the health requirements of the population are and how they should be met. At the same time, demand is growing for value for money and for accountability to the public for decisions in health policy and practice. Questions of ethics that arise in health policy and practice have hitherto been a preoccupation normally restricted to governments, associations of health professionals and certain other groups such as lawyers, philosophers and theologians. As the concept of health policy has widened to include lifestyle and environmental issues, the number of disciplines and professions that contribute to health policy formulation has grown. The complexity of many health policy issues, their ethical implications and the intense concern they arouse have grown to the point where they can no longer be effectively dealt with through traditional institutions or delegated by government and society to the professionals immediately concerned.

This has been pointedly demonstrated by the AIDS epidemic, which has raised a combination of ethical and moral issues that affect the community, people with HIV and AIDS, and health care providers. Many such issues touch basic individual and collective human rights: the right of HIV-infected women to bear children, the protection against discrimination of HIV-infected people and whole groups perceived to be at risk of infection, mandatory reporting and conditions of screening, measures to protect health personnel and their patients, and the conditions under which AIDS research is carried out *(39,40)*.

Issues of ethics and conflicts of value systems that arise in deciding on health action fall into three categories: health policy, the rights of individuals and groups of patients, and specific health care interventions.

Ethics and health policy   In broad terms, the health policy issues are of two sorts: those concerned with human rights and those involving the allocation of public funds for health. The more traditional concerns have had to do with balancing the rights of the individual with the protection of the community through public order and public health. Examples include taking violently disturbed individuals into custody, notifying the authorities about cases of diseases of public health concern, and protecting people against infectious diseases through mandatory immunization.

A new set of issues has emerged as the concept of health promotion has broadened to take more account of more issues of lifestyle and behaviour. For example, debate about the appropriateness of government regulations on the mandatory wearing of seat-belts has been extensive. Other issues include environmental restrictions on smoking, the use of high taxes to discourage some forms of consumption, and restrictions on the production and marketing of tobacco, alcohol and additives.

Two factors have led to the increasing complexity and prominence of ethical issues in deciding how to allocate human, technical and financial resources for health. One is the broadening concept of health policy, and the other is the growth of extremely expensive technology, which can increasingly be used to save or prolong life, usually for a very small number of people and for a relatively short period of time. The major policy choices concern the apportionment of expenditure between health promotion and disease prevention or treatment and care, between proven or experimental technologies and therapies, between active treatment or supportive care, and among various research and development priorities.

The complex array of alternatives has in practice meant more rationing of resources. The serious political and ethical consequences are evident from debates about human organ transplantation, the development of new medical technology, and investment in pollution control and safety in the workplace. Whatever political judgement may be made in a given situation about the allocation of resources, it would be ethically indefensible to fund inappropriate or ineffective, expensive technologies by diverting resources away from primary care development, from innovative strategies for health promotion and disease prevention, or from treatments of proven effectiveness.

Ethics and the consumer of health services The second category of ethical issues involves people's rights when using the health care system. It is now recognized that people have the right to life-saving and life-sustaining care without financial, social or physical barriers. It is widely accepted that the patient and, in many cases, his or her family should be full partners in treatment and care processes and bring their knowledge, values and priorities to bear on the decisions made. But this new understanding of the patient's role generates new demands. One is the right to information about the immediate benefits and risks of the treatment being used and the alternative therapies that may be available. Associated with this is the patient's right to give informed consent to treatment, as well as the demand for the health care provider to be more accountable. On the other hand, exercising the right to be given information can place an additional emotional and intellectual burden on some patients that may harm their medical condition. Doctors need training to help them assess a patient's capacity to carry that burden, support that patient in contemplating any decision he or she should make, and decide what action ethically to take when they conclude that a patient cannot carry the burden without harm.

Ethics and intervention A third ethical concern is the potential for intervention at key points in the life cycle, especially reproduction, perinatal care and the prolongation of life, and the conditions under which research may be conducted. These issues become increasingly critical as technology can save and prolong life in situations where death would otherwise occur. These advances are challenging traditional understandings of the nature of life and the boundaries of appropriate human intervention in life and death.

Reproductive issues concern contraceptive technology, abortion, *in vitro* fertilization and the manipulation of gene material. Concerns about perinatal treatment focus on the appropriateness of saving the lives of premature infants who are known to have major birth defects, regardless of the long-term consequences for the quality of life of the children, for the wellbeing of their families and for those who provide and will pay for their care. The concern with technology and treatment that prolong the lives of older people is that a marginal increase in longevity (adding years to life) may be achieved at the cost of considerable suffering or distress and without any benefit of adding health to life and life to years.

Ethics and research   The ethics of health research are gaining greater prominence as decisions on health policy and action are increasingly required to be based on scientific evidence. One concern is that the acquisition of knowledge becomes a driving force in treatment decisions, and active treatment is given higher priority than either care or prevention. These are prominent concerns in cancer treatment and care. Questions are being raised about how research priorities are set and what capacity research institutions have to deal with these emerging questions.

Suggested solutions   The approaches adopted to address ethics, and associated value questions,

in health action and research must be based on political decisions made after wide public discussion and political debate. The arrangements made will depend on a country's political systems, cultural traditions, constitutional arrangements and organizational structures. Some countries have found it useful to express or support these in appropriate laws and regulations. Whatever the arrangements used, questions must be dealt with in an equitable, broad, transparent and balanced manner.

Any policies on health and ethics should take full account of the relevant articles in the United Nations Universal Declaration of Human Rights, of other internationally recognized conventions in the field of human rights and bioethics, and of the protection of the individual contained in the constitutions of Member States. Considerations of equity and of access to the prerequisites for health will also need to be addressed. In dealing with such questions, the legitimate interests and rights of the individual and of particular groups of people should be balanced with the good of the community.

Issues in bioethics, including the implications of research involving human subjects, have been receiving increasing attention. The Council of Europe has reviewed a number of specific issues and has reached consensus on respect for human dignity, recognition of the inviolability of the human body, avoidance of commercial profiteering in the field of biomedicine, and the principle of self determination of the individual.

Ethics and accountability   A great deal of progress can be made in ethical issues if accountability to the public can be established as a guiding principle for decisions made about health action. This means that the people who decide on policy and practice in any area of health development may have their decisions publicly examined in terms of their health consequences, with the possibility of corrective action being taken. Processes for achieving accountability and forms of corrective action can vary widely, depending on national and local circumstances. The principle of accountability applies broadly to decisions that affect health care, environmental protection, lifestyles, equity and the prerequisites for health.

Ensuring open debate   Countries have found it useful to have an agreed set of structures and processes for obtaining advice and facilitating public discussion in a representative manner. All institutions established to address ethical issues must have mandates and working methods that are clearly stated. While these bodies will reflect the particular political, cultural and other features of the country, three characteristics have been found to be beneficial.

First, they should be independent in the sense that they are protected from undue influence from political, professional, commercial or religious interests. This can be achieved by giving these bodies a high degree of autonomy when setting their agendas, when deciding whose opinions to take into account and what basis of knowledge and opinion to accept, and when publishing their investigations and conclusions.

Second, they should allow the public to participate in their activities, thus conducting their business in an open, transparent and accountable manner.

Third, their membership and the manner in which they conduct their activities should be representative. This may mean that membership includes individuals who represent the public interest, and that structures and processes are adopted that ensure that particular interests are accommodated and balanced representation is achieved. In countries with well established self-governing bodies of providers and other health care partners that address ethical issues as part of their overall mandate, it has been found useful to institute transparent mechanisms for dialogue between the parties. In every case, the procedures established should ensure that all parties affected by deliberations on ethical and related issues have an opportunity to be heard and involved in those deliberations.

The strategy for addressing ethical issues must be able to involve broad sections of the public, including particular interest groups, in an informed process of discussion. This is most likely to succeed if the strategy is based on two-way communication. The people who have an interest in any issue, such as consumer and self-help groups, professional associations and health researchers, should have an opportunity to contribute what they consider to be their legitimate points of view and knowledge about it. At the same time, the mass media and others in a position to contribute to discussions should also be actively engaged in the communications process.

Leadership and responsibility of the health care professional   A strategy of participation and openness also increases knowledge and awareness among the public, politicians and decision-makers. Physicians and other health care providers have traditionally taken the lead in advocating what they consider to be the best courses of action for their patients and the appropriate policies for the settings in which they work. They should continue to play their leadership role, but also recognize that they work in a wide social and political framework containing many other players. They should be conscious of their role in making decisions about policy and practice, keep under continuous review their codes of practice and revise them as new circumstances demand. Innovative approaches to training are clearly needed to address ethical issues as a part of the education of all health professionals. This means developing training programmes that integrate moral and philosophical concepts with biomedical and other relevant scientific knowledge and with the development of technical skills in ways that strengthen the professional competence of the practitioner.

Ethics and trade   Finally, goods and services with both good and bad influences on health are becoming increasingly standardized and freely traded across international boundaries. This challenges the international community to pay greater attention to health and ethics associated with economic trade and development.

References

1. WHITEHEAD, M. *The concepts and principles of equity and health.* Copenhagen, WHO Regional Office for Europe, 1990 (document EUR/ICP/RPD 414).
2. HERMAN, R. *The European scientific community.* Harlow, Longman Group, 1986.
3. *Implementation of the global strategy for health for all by the year 2000, second evaluation: eighth report on the world health situation. Volume 5. European Region.* Copenhagen, WHO Regional Office for Europe, 1993 (WHO Regional Publications, European Series, No. 52).
4. *Research policies for health for all.* Copenhagen, WHO Regional Office for Europe, 1988 (European Health for All Series, No. 2).
5. *Priority research for health for all.* Copenhagen, WHO Regional Office for Europe, 1988 (European Health for All Series, No. 3).
6. DAVIES, A.M. & MANSOURIAN, B., ED. *Research strategies for health.* Lewiston, NY, Hogrefe & Huber, 1992.
7. VUORI, H. Health for all through research. *Arhiv za higijenu rada i toksikologiju,* **42**: 1 – 11 (1991).
8. VUORI, H. Health for all through research on primary health care. *Scandinavian journal of primary health care,* **10**: 3 – 6 (1992).
9. DEKKER, E. & VAN DER WERFF, A., ED. *Policies for health in European countries with pluralistic systems.* Houten, Bohn Stafleu Van Loghum, 1990.
10. *Consultation of countries with national health for all policy documents*: report on a WHO meeting. Copenhagen, WHO Regional Office for Europe, 1990 (document EUR/ICP/MPN 040).
11. *The process of health policy development*: report of a working group on the development of subnational policies for health. Copenhagen, WHO Regional Office for Europe, 1992 (document EUR/ICP/HSC 418).
12. *Evaluation of the strategy for health for all by the year 2000. Seventh report on the world health situation. Vol. 5. European Region.* Copenhagen, WHO Regional Office for Europe, 1986.
13. *Monitoring of the strategy for health for all by the year 2000. Part 1: the situation in the European Region, 1987/1988.* Copenhagen, WHO Regional Office for Europe, 1989 (document EUR/HST/89.1).
14. *Monitoring of the strategy for health for all by the year 2000. Part 2: monitoring by country, 1988/1989.* Copenhagen, WHO Regional Office for Europe, 1989 (document EUR/ICP/EXM 021).

15. TAKET, A.R., ED. *Making partners: intersectoral action for health*: proceedings and outcome of a joint working group on intersectoral action for health. The Hague, Ministry of Welfare, Health and Cultural Affairs, 1990.

16. *Health for all policy in Finland: WHO health policy review*. Copenhagen, WHO Regional Office for Europe, 1991 (document EUR/FIN/HSC 410).

17. VUORI, H. & HASTINGS, J., ED. *Patterns of community participation in primary health care*. Copenhagen, WHO Regional Office for Europe, 1984 (document EUR/ICP/PHC 301/s01).

18. BENGOA, R. & HUNTER, D.J., ED. *New directions in managing health care*. Proceedings and outcome of a working group on new approaches to managing health services. Leeds, Nuffield Institute for Health Services Studies, 1991.

19. ARTUNDO, C. ET AL., ED. *Health care reforms in Europe*. Proceedings of the first meeting of the Working Party. Copenhagen, WHO Regional Office for Europe, 1993 (document EUR/ICP/PHC 210(B)).

20. *Health monitoring systems and epidemiology as a basis for health policy decisions*: report on a WHO Symposium. Copenhagen, WHO Regional Office for Europe, 1990 (document EUR/ICP/HST 123).

21. *European HFA information strategy*. Copenhagen, WHO Regional Office for Europe, 1990 (document EUR/RC40/11).

22. *Development of guidelines for reports on public health*: report on a WHO Working Group. Copenhagen, WHO Regional Office for Europe, 1991 (document EUR/ICP/HSC 016).

23. *Common methods and instruments for health interview surveys*: report on the Second WHO Consultation. Copenhagen, WHO Regional Office for Europe, 1991 (document EUR/ICP/HST 124).

24. BANKOWSKI, Z. & MEJIA, A., ED. *Health manpower out of balance: conflicts and prospects*. Conference papers, conclusions and recommendations: XX CIOMS Conference. Geneva, CIOMS, 1987.

25. ENGEL, C.E. ET AL. *Continuing education for change*. Copenhagen, WHO Regional Office for Europe, 1990 (WHO Regional Publications, European Series, No. 28).

26. *Future developments in the areas of human resources policies, planning and management*: report on an informal consultation. Geneva, World Health Organization, 1991 (document HRH/91.1).

27. BERG, B. & OSTERGREN, B. *Innovations and innovation processes in higher education*. Stockholm, National Board of Universities and Colleges, 1977.

28. GARCIA-BARBERO, M. A methodological framework for translating health for all targets into educational programmes. *In*: Menu, J.P. & Garcia-Barbero, M., ed. *Health manpower education for health for all: issues to be considered*. Proceedings of a consultation held in Venice, 4 – 8 December 1989. Milan, Franco-Angeli, 1991.

29. BURY, J. Integrating basic HFA themes into health personnel education. *In*: Menu, J.P. & Garcia-Barbero, M., ed. *Health manpower education for health for all: issues to be considered*. Proceedings of a consultation held in Venice, 4 – 8 December 1989. Milan, Franco-Angeli, 1991.

30. WHO Technical Report Series, No. 769, 1988 (*Learning together to work together for health*: report of a WHO Study Group on Multiprofessional Education of Health Personnel: the Team Approach).

31. WORLD FEDERATION FOR MEDICAL EDUCATION. The Edinburgh declaration. *Medical education*, **22**: 481 – 482 (1988).

32. *Ministerial consultation for medical education in Europe*: report on a WHO meeting. Copenhagen, WHO Regional Office for Europe, 1989 (document EUR/ICP/HMD 115(S)).

33. *European Conference on Nursing*: report on a WHO meeting. Copenhagen, WHO Regional Office for Europe, 1989.

34. *Investment in health*. Proceedings of the International Conference on Health Promotion, Bonn, 17 – 19 December 1990. Bonn, Wissenschaftliches Institut der Ärzte Deutschlands, 1990 (document EUR 14281 EN).

35. *The role of the media in AIDS prevention and control*: report on a WHO Workshop. Copenhagen, WHO Regional Office for Europe, 1991 (document EUR/ICP/GPA 053).

36. *AIDS service organizations into the 1990s: people's needs and the best response*: report on a WHO Workshop. Copenhagen, WHO Regional Office for Europe, 1991 (document EUR/ICP/GPA 095).

37. ASHTON, J. ET AL. Healthy Cities: WHO's new public health initiative. *Health promotion*, **1**(3): 319 – 324 (1986).

38. KICKBUSCH, I. Healthy Cities: a working project and a growing movement. *Health promotion*, **4**(2): 77 – 82 (1989).

39. *HIV/AIDS in the context of public health and human rights*: report of a Pan-European Consultation. London, International Association of Rights and Humanity, 1991.

40. *Health legislation and ethics in the field of AIDS and HIV infection*: report on an International Consultation. Oslo, Directorate of Health, 1988.

8

Conclusions

Health for all is a challenging goal for the Region as a whole and for each of its Member States. Through their resolutions in the World Health Assembly and the WHO Regional Committee for Europe, all Member States have accepted the duty and responsibility of taking the action necessary to ensure the attainment of health for all. This book provides a framework for intensifying such action. It suggests the changes and interventions needed to improve people's health and the support that these require.

The experience gained since the first set of regional targets was adopted has demonstrated the soundness and relevance of the concepts and approaches on which health for all is based. A new direction has been set for health development in the European Region. Major improvements in terms of longer life and better health have been accompanied by increasing knowledge about programmes and practices that work. Countries have benefited not just in the immediate health field but in many other areas, through the adoption of policies that reflect the principles and strategies of health for all.

Unsolved problems remain, however, that set the agenda for the rest of this decade. Progress in the acceptance of health for all policies has been greater than achievements in implementing them. The need for leadership and good management has become more pronounced as health promotion and environmental protection play a stronger role and countries move increasingly towards pluralistic systems.

The main emphasis of the updated European health for all policy, and the revised targets described in this book, is on implementation. It calls for greater efforts in health promotion, disease prevention, environmental health, appropriate care and health development support. It is about action, partnership and innovation at the international, country, regional and local levels. It seeks new ways of involving and mobilizing a large number of individuals as well as public, private and voluntary bodies in all sectors of society. It aims to turn policy intentions into successful outcomes that will produce healthier populations, bringing not just basic benefits but the best quality achievements possible. It encourages policy-makers to employ strategies that will reduce, and where possible eliminate, inequalities in health, and make the best use of society's resources to maximize health potential.

Action does not mean tackling the health for all targets one by one. Rather, the challenge is to combine components related to different targets into cohesive programmes of action. Each component can stimulate the interests of the public, private and voluntary sectors at the local, national and international levels, giving them the incentive to make significant progress towards health for all.

The most relevant components and the most important interactions will differ according to each particular situation, in social, cultural, economic and political terms. The heart of the health for all approach is to encourage local, regional, national or international action that is flexible, adaptive and responsive.

As an illustration, a programme of action on tobacco, which is the single largest cause of preventable death, disability and disease in the Region, could involve components from many different targets, as shown in the table.

Action programme on tobacco:
potential components relating to different targets

Programme component	Related target(s)
Working with groups in society most vulnerable to tobacco use	1
Increasing the health potential of groups, communities and individuals by reducing the social attractiveness of tobacco	2
Reducing cancer, cardiovascular diseases and chronic obstructive lung disease caused by smoking	4
Increasing the quality of life of elderly people by reducing their disability from smoking-related diseases and by increasing their disposable income for travel, cultural events and other forms of participation in social life	6
Championing nonsmoking as an the "in-thing" among children and youth	7
Combating the marketing of tobacco to women by presenting smoke-free living as having a positive value in the family and society	8

Programme component	Related target(s)
Promoting nonsmoking in cardiovascular disease and cancer control programmes in community and clinical settings	9,10
Presenting smoke-free living as having a positive value in lifestyle programmes, supported by healthy public policy in other sectors; ensuring that the choice of either tobacco or health is a key part of health education and training	13 – 17
Creating healthier environments free from tobacco pollution in enclosed spaces at work, in public places and at home	19 – 21
Protecting people at work from the use of tobacco, which is an obstacle to health and quality of life, a fire hazard and a workplace pollutant	25
Procuring health service resources and appropriate technology for efficient programmes of education about tobacco or health, and the development of the skills necessary for community health promotion	27 – 31
Ensuring smoke-free health institutions and encouraging health service staff, as important role models, to support tobacco or health programmes in their public lives	28 – 30
Promoting evaluation and research linked to the action programme on tobacco, to test and improve its effectiveness, efficiency and accessibility to the whole community	32
Developing a process of implementation and management appropriate to this high priority issue in the Region	33,34
Ensuring the availability and efficient use of monitoring information on smoking knowledge, attitudes and behaviour, public policy provision, and the pattern and impact of tobacco-related disease	35
Establishing a programme of recruitment, training and deployment of key human resources in the public, private and voluntary sectors for the promotion and fulfilment of the action programme on tobacco	36
Securing the participation and cooperation of the community and key political, professional, social and cultural groups, particularly the mass media, to support the programme in an effective and timely way	37
Justifying the ethics of supporting the rights of nonsmokers	38

Action for health for all is the responsibility of the entire community. Models of good practice have developed in different target areas in many parts of the Region and, in the last few years, have also been widely applied at the local level. The economic and political changes that are taking place throughout the Region offer both a challenge and an opportunity to develop new structures for mutual inspiration, practical cooperation and shared decision-making.

Health authorities in countries will continue to lead the process of health for all, supported by the commitment of a large number of professional and other groups. Collectively, they must ensure that the WHO Regional Committee for Europe can continue to play its key role in stimulating health for all development, further developing the common health policy, monitoring its implementation, and evaluating its effectiveness in achieving the regional targets. The Regional Committee must also ensure that the inspiration, guidance and coordination of regional health work by the WHO Regional Office for Europe are maintained. The resources of the Regional Office should support the implementation and development of health for all strategies in individual countries and in the Region as a whole.

The European Region has the people, the knowledge and the resources that are needed to attain the regional targets, and the will to bring these forces to bear on the prevailing problems. Each step made together will bring countries closer to health for all. By jointly making the commitment to a regional health for all policy and by setting clear targets, the Member States of the Region have created a broad movement that fosters better understanding among nations and will leave a legacy of value beyond our time.

Annex 1

Revision of the targets for health for all

This annex summarizes the nature and extent of changes to the targets (see table), by comparing those in this book with those set out in the original book, *Targets for health for all* (European Health for All Series, No. 1, 1985).

Within the targets on health outcome (targets 1 – 12) the major changes are to targets 6 – 8. The updated targets have been refocused to deal with the health of different population groups: target 6 now focuses on the elderly, target 7 on children and young people, and target 8 on women. In each case the original target is retained as a component of the updated target, but the updated targets have a much broader scope and positively and comprehensively emphasize the health of the population group concerned. The scope of target 12 has also been widened to deal with mental disorders and the quality of life of people with such disorders, as well as with suicide and attempted suicide.

There are two major changes to the targets on lifestyles and health (13 – 17). The first of these is target 14, which has a new focus on the development of opportunities for health promotion in the

settings of daily life. The second is a reorganization of the material covered in targets 16 and 17. The revised target 16 is concerned with healthy patterns of living (in contrast to its original emphasis on individuals and behaviour). The reduction of tobacco use is now a part of target 17, which calls for controlling the health-damaging consumption of tobacco, alcohol and psychoactive drugs.

The targets on creating healthy environments (18 – 25) remain largely unchanged. In two cases the scope of the target has been widened. Target 23 now includes soil pollution and the disposal of municipal waste as well as hazardous waste, while target 25 has been widened to include the promotion of health and wellbeing at work.

The reorganization of subject matter among the targets on appropriate care (26 – 31) has allowed the formulation of two substantially new targets. Target 29, now entitled "Hospital care", deals with secondary and tertiary care in support of primary health care. Target 30 concerns the provision of appropriate services to people requiring long-term care and support (developed from part of original

Changes in the targets

Target number	Original title	Revised title	Extent of revision
1	Reducing the differences	Equity in health	None
2	Developing health potential	Health and quality of life	None
3	Better opportunities for the disabled	Better opportunities for people with disabilities	None
4	Reducing disease and disability	Reducing chronic disease	Minor changes
5	Elimination of specific diseases	Reducing communicable disease	Minor changes
6	Life expectancy at birth	Healthy aging	Substantially different; revised to cover the elderly as a population group
7	Infant mortality	Health of children and young people	Substantially different; revised to cover children and young people as a population group
8	Maternal mortality	Health of women	Substantially different; revised to cover women as a population group
9	Diseases of the circulation	Reducing cardiovascular disease	Minor changes
10	Cancer	Controlling cancer	Minor changes
11	Accidents	Accidents	Minor changes
12	Suicide	Reducing mental disorders and suicide	Minor changes
13	Healthy public policy	Healthy public policy	Minor changes
14	Social support systems	Settings for health promotion	Refocused on the development of opportunities for health promotion in particular settings
15	Knowledge and motivation for healthy behaviour	Health competence	Minor changes
16	Positive health behaviour	Healthy living	Minor changes
17	Health-damaging behaviour	Tobacco, alcohol and psychoactive drugs	Refocused on controlling the production and consumption of tobacco, alcohol and psychoactive drugs
18	Multisectoral policies	Policy on environment and health	Minor changes
19	Monitoring and control mechanisms	Environmental health management	Minor changes
20	Control of water pollution	Water quality	Minor changes

Target number	Original title	Revised title	Extent of revision
21	Control of air pollution	Air quality	Minor changes
22	Food safety	Food quality and safety	Minor changes
23	Control of hazardous wastes	Waste management and soil pollution	Widened to include soil pollution and disposal of municipal waste
24	Human settlements and housing	Human ecology and settlements	Minor changes
25	Working environment	Health of people at work	Widened to include health initiatives at the workplace that focus on lifestyle
26	A system based on primary health care	Health service policy	Minor changes
27	Rational and preferential distribution of resources	Health service resources and management	Minor changes
28	Content of primary health care	Primary health care	Minor changes; takes in elements from original targets 29 and 30
29	Providers of primary health care	Hospital care	Substantially different; focuses on secondary and tertiary care in support of primary care
30	Coordination of community resources	Community services to meet special needs	Substantially different; incorporates part of original target 28
31	Ensuring quality of care	Quality of care and appropriate technology	Substantially different; widened to include technology
32	Research strategies	Health research and development	Minor changes
33	Policies for health for all	Health for all policy development	Minor changes
34	Planning and resource allocation	Managing health for all development	Minor changes
35	Health information systems	Health information support	Minor changes
36	Planning, education and use of health personnel	Developing human resources for health	Widened to include other sectors as well as health
37	Education of personnel in other sectors	Partners for health	Substantially different
38	Appropriate health technology	Health and ethics	New

target 28). The original targets 29 and 30 (on the content and providers of primary health care, respectively) are now dealt with as part of updated target 28 on primary health care. Finally, target 31 now covers both the quality of care (original target 31) and appropriate technology (original target 38).

The last seven targets (32 – 38) deal with health for all development. Target 36, on education and train-ing, has been widened and now deals not just with health workers but personnel in all sectors (taking in the subjects covered by original target 37). The updated target 37 is completely refocused on mobilizing partners and facilitating widespread cooperation and participation in health for all development. Updated target 38 on health and ethics is completely new, and deals with mechanisms to strengthen ethical considerations in decisions relating to health.

Indicators for monitoring progress towards health for all in the WHO European Region

This annex sets out the statistical indicators for use with the revised targets. The WHO Regional Committee for Europe approved this list of indicators in 1991, along with the updated regional targets for health for all and the revised plan of action and major milestones for implementation of the regional strategy.

During the latest evaluation of progress towards health for all, carried out in 1990 – 1991, narrative situation assessments were introduced to be used as a guide in reporting on the aspects of the targets that could not be covered adequately by statistical indicators. Such assessments will be adapted to cover all the components of each of the revised target statements in future evaluation and monitoring exercises. Specific formulations and definitions of the set of indicators and narrative situation assessments for use in the next monitoring exercise are to be available for review at the forty-third session of the Regional Committee.

For a number of the proposed new or revised statistical indicators, further work is required before specific recommendations can be made on suitable standardized measurement instruments for use in future monitoring and evaluation exercises. The indicators concerned are those on the quality of life (targets 2, 3, 6, 9, 10 and 12), healthy life expectancy (target 2), injury or disability resulting from accidents (target 11), mental health (target 12), and adequate nutrition and exercise (target 16). Specific recommendations in each of these areas will be put before the Regional Committee at the earliest opportunity, for incorporation in the list of indicators. Member States will be welcome to report on the results of specific surveys or studies that include the areas concerned.

Data for some indicators can be collated from an international source or sources. In such cases, Member States will not have to supply data on these indicators during monitoring and evaluation exercises. The notes in the indicator list show where such common sources will be used.

List of indicators

Target		Regional indicators		
No.	Title	No.	Description	Comment
1	Equity in health	1.1	Differences in health status between countries	Data from health status indicators listed below for targets 2 – 12 will be used.
		1.2	Differences in health status within countries	No detailed statistical indicators can be specified, since Member States are expected to differ in the subgroups that can be identified, and in the most relevant subgroups, as well as in the measures of health status (apart from mortality) that are available. Subgroups could be defined by: social class, occupational group, educational level, income level, ethnic/cultural origin or identification,and region/ district of residence. Sources could be routine or special surveys/studies. At the least, all countries are likely to be able to report mortality by geographical division such as district/region or urban/rural area.
2	Health and quality of life	2.2	Assessment of perceived health	
		2.5	Proportion of unemployed persons	Source will be ILO publications.
		2.6	Assessment of social health and support	
		2.7	Assessment of quality of life	Although a variety of approaches and measurement instruments have been developed for assessing the quality of life, standardized instruments cannot yet be recommended for use throughout the Region. Clear working definitions of quality of life and review of the instruments available are required before specific recommendations can be formulated.
		2.8	Healthy life expectancy: indices linking life tables with functional aspects of health	Standard methods of calculation cannot yet be recommended for use throughout the Region. Specific recommendations will be submitted to the Regional Committee for approval at the earliest possible opportunity.
3	Better opportunities for people with disabilities	3.2	Percentage of disabled persons of working age engaged in regular occupational activities	

Target		Regional indicators		
No.	Title	No.	Description	Comment
3	Better opportunities for people with disabilities	3.3	Assessment of quality of life for people with disabilities	See comments on the assessment of quality of life under target 2.
4	Reducing chronic disease	4.1	Number of days of temporary disability per person per year, by age and sex	Data for indicators 4.1, 4.2, 4.5 and 4.6 on people over 65 years of age, where they can be supplied, will also be relevant to target 6.
		4.2	Percentage of the population experiencing different levels of long-term disability, by age and sex	Results obtained from population surveys and from surveys of disabled people will also be relevant to targets 2 and 3, respectively.
		4.3	Incidence of: – tuberculosis (010-018)[a] – viral hepatitis (070) – pertussis (033) – syphilis (090-097) – gonococcal infections (098) – other venereal diseases (099) – AIDS (279.5)	Data will be collated from those already reported to WHO and its collaborating centres. Data on AIDS will also be relevant to target 5.
		4.5	Disability-free life expectancy at birth and at ages 1, 15, 45 and 65 years, by sex	The Sullivan method may be used: details are given in *World health statistics quarterly*, **42**(3): 148 (1989). Values for disability-free life expectancy at age 65 years will also be used in connection with target 6.
		4.6	Incidence and prevalence of selected chronic conditions: all ages, by sex; people aged 65 years and over, by sex	The most suitable conditions for reporting may be neoplasms (information from registries), mental disorders, diseases of the circulatory system, diseases of the musculoskeletal system, chronic diseases of the respiratory system and diabetes. For people aged 65 years and over, locomotor and sensory disorders and senile dementia are also relevant. Data for the population aged 65 years and over will also be used in connection with target 6.

[a] Numbers in brackets are rubrics of ICD-9.

Target		Regional indicators		
No.	Title	No.	Description	Comment
4	Reducing chronic disease	4.7	Oral health: - average number of decayed, missing or filled teeth at 12 years - average number of missing teeth per person in age group 35 – 44 years	Data from the Regional Office oral health information system will usually be used.
		4.9	Long-term incapacity for work by age and sex	
5	Reducing communicable disease	5.1	Number of cases of: - measles (055) - acute poliomyelitis (045) - tetanus (037) - neonatal tetanus (771.3) - congenital rubella (771.0) - diphtheria (032) - congenital syphilis (090) - indigenous malaria (084) - mumps (072)	Data will usually be taken from existing notification systems.
		5.2	Mortality rates in children under 5 years of age from: - pneumonia (480-486) - diarrhoeal disease (001-009)	Source will be routinely reported mortality data.
		5.3	Estimates of rates of transmission of HIV infection	
		5.4	Estimates of the incidence of severe complications associated with major sexually transmitted diseases	
6	Healthy aging	6.1	Life expectancy at birth, by sex, in all identifiable subgroups	The revised target focuses on the reduction of variations in life expectancy within countries. Member States are expected to differ in the subgroups that can be identified, and in the most relevant subgroups. Possibilities for reporting include differences between social classes, occupational groups, educational levels, income levels, ethnic/cultural origin or identification, and region/district of residence.

Target		Regional indicators		
No.	Title	No.	Description	Comment
6	Healthy aging	6.2	Life expectancy at ages 1, 15, 45 and 65 years, by sex	Source will be routinely reported mortality data.
		6.3	Number of years of life lost as a result of death occurring before the age of 65 years	Source will be routinely reported mortality data.
		6.4	Probability of dying before 5 years of age in all identifiable subgroups	
		6.5	Assessment of quality of life for those aged 65 years and over	See comments on the assessment of quality of life under target 2.
7	Health of children and young people	7.1	Infant mortality rates, including neonatal and postneonatal mortality rates, in all identifiable subgroups	The revised target focuses on reducing variations in infant mortality within countries. Member States are expected to differ in the subgroups that can be identified, and in the most relevant subgroups. Possibilities for reporting include differences between social classes, occupational groups, educational levels, income levels, ethnic/cultural origin or identification, and region/district of residence. In order to avoid problems due to small numbers of events, it may be necessary to calculate rates over several years. Data from indicators 11.1, 11.2, 16.5, 16.6, 28.5 and 28.6 will also be relevant to this target.
		7.4	Perinatal mortality rate	
		7.5	Proportion of children abused, by age and sex	Comprehensive data may not be readily available. Interpretation of trends is particularly difficult owing to changes in reporting levels, recording practices, etc. (which are affected by the treatment given and services offered to children who disclose abuse), as well as to changes in actual incidence. Thus, trends in individual countries will have to be examined against the information given on these other factors in the narrative situation assessments and/or other sources.

Target		Regional indicators		
No.	Title	No.	Description	Comment
8	Health of women	8.1	Maternal mortality rates in all identifiable subgroups	The revised target focuses on the reduction of variations in maternal mortality within countries. Member States are expected to differ in the subgroups that can be identified, and in the most relevant subgroups. Possibilities for reporting include differences between social classes, occupational groups, educational levels, income levels, ethnic/cultural origin or identification, and region/district of residence. Since maternal deaths are often extremely few in any one year, rates may be reported over several years to avoid problems due to small numbers of events.
		8.2	Sex differences in selected social indicators such as income, education and employment	
		8.3	Incidence or prevalence of pelvic inflammatory disease	Comprehensive data related to indicators 8.3 to 8.6 may not be readily available, in which case sources will be special surveys or studies where available.
		8.4	Rate of Caesarean section in childbirth	
		8.5	Incidence of unplanned pregnancies, by age	
		8.6	Percentage of women having access to adequate contraceptive services	
		8.7	Incidence of rape, attempted rape and sexual assault	Comprehensive data may not be readily available. Interpretation of trends is particularly difficult owing to changes in reporting levels, recording practices, etc. (which are affected by the treatment given and services offered to women who report a rape or sexual assault) as well as to changes in actual incidence. Thus trends in individual countries will have to be examined against the information given on these other factors in the narrative situation assessments.

Target		Regional indicators		
No.	Title	No.	Description	Comment
8	Health of women	8.8	Number of households consisting of one adult female plus dependents (children and/or dependent adults), and as a percentage of the total number of households	This is a suitable, although not perfect, proxy measure for multiple burdens on women. It should be noted that this is usually *not* the same as the number of households headed by women.
			The information supplied for indicators on health status in targets 1 – 7 and 9 – 12, where the information is provided separately for women, will also be relevant to this target. Indicator 28.5 will also be relevant.	
9	Reducing cardiovascular disease	9.1	Mortality rates, by sex and age, from diseases of the circulatory system (390-459)	Source will be routinely reported mortality data.
		9.2	Mortality rates, by sex and age, from ischaemic heart disease (410-414)	Source will be routinely reported mortality data.
		9.3	Mortality rates, by sex and age, from cerebro-vascular diseases (430-438)	Source will be routinely reported mortality data.
		9.4	Incidence of ischaemic heart disease (410-414)	
		9.5	Incidence of cerebro-vascular diseases (430-438)	
		9.6	Assessment of quality of life for people with cardiovascular disease	See comments on the assessment of quality of life under target 2.
		9.7	Serum cholesterol and blood pressure levels, by age and sex	Data can be made available from population surveys or international projects such as MONICA.
			As in the case of many chronic diseases, indicators 16.7, 16.10 and 17.10 will also be relevant to this target.	

Target		Regional indicators		
No.	Title	No.	Description	Comment
10	Controlling cancer	10.1	Mortality rates, by sex and age, from malignant neoplasms (140-208)	Source will be routinely reported mortality data.
		10.2	Mortality rates, by sex and age, from malignant neoplasms of the trachea, bronchus and lung (162)	Source will be routinely reported mortality data.
		10.3	Mortality rates, by sex and age, from malignant neoplasms of the cervix uteri (180)	Source will be routinely reported mortality data.
		10.4	Incidence of malignant neoplasms of the cervix uteri (180)	
		10.5	Mortality rates, by age, from malignant neoplasms of the female breast (174)	Source will be routinely reported mortality data.
		10.6	Incidence of malignant neoplasms of the female breast (174)	
		10.7	Mortality rates, by sex and age, from malignant neoplasms of the colon and rectum (153-154)	Source will be routinely reported mortality data.
		10.8	Assessment of quality of life for people with cancer	See comments on the assessment of quality of life under target 2.
11	Accidents	11.1	Mortality rates, by sex and age, from external causes of injury and poisoning (E800-E949)	Source will be routinely reported mortality data.
		11.2	Mortality rates, by sex and age, from motor vehicle traffic accidents (E810-E819)	Source will be routinely reported mortality data.

Target		Regional indicators		
No.	**Title**	**No.**	**Description**	**Comment**
11	Accidents	11.3	Occurrence of road traffic accidents leading to personal injury	Information from ECE publications will be used.
		11.4	Accidents in the home due to poisoning and other factors	
		11.5	Work-related accidents leading to personal injury	Data from ILO publications will be used.
		11.6	Incidence of injury or disability resulting from accidents, preferably disaggregated by type of accident (traffic, home, occupational, sports and leisure)	Specific recommendations will be submitted to the Regional Committee for approval at the earliest possible opportunity.
12	Reducing mental disorders and suicide	12.1	Mortality rates, by sex and age, from suicide and self-inflicted injury (E950-E959)	Source will be routinely reported mortality data.
		12.2	Assessment of quality of life for people with mental disorders	See comments on the assessment of quality of life under target 2.
		12.3	Mental health	Further work is required to review the possibility of standardizing measurement and reporting. Specific recommendations will be submitted to the Regional Committee for approval at the earliest possible opportunity.
13	Healthy public policy		No statistical indicators; narrative situation assessment only.	
14	Settings for health promotion		No statistical indicators; narrative situation assessment only.	
15	Health competence	15.2	Adult literacy rate by sex, in all identifiable subgroups	Data from UNESCO publications will be used for indicators 15.2 and 15.5.
		15.5	Proportion of the population having reached various educational levels, by age group	

Target		Regional indicators		
No.	Title	No.	Description	Comment
16	Healthy living	16.3	Percentage of total energy intake from fat and from protein	Food balance sheet data from FAO will be used.
		16.4	Percentage of neonates having a birth weight of at least 2500 g	Where available, disaggregation by sex, urban and rural areas and/or by geographical or administrative subdivisions and/or by defined socioeconomic groups (such as level of mother's education) will also be relevant.
		16.5	Percentage of children with acceptable weight for age and/or weight for height	
		16.6	Percentage of children breastfed at six weeks, three months and six months of age	
		16.7	"Energy expenditure patterns", by age, sex and socioeconomic groups: – total daily energy expenditure – daily energy expenditure for physical leisure activities – energy expenditure for physical leisure activities of higher intensity	
		16.10	Distribution of body mass index by age and sex, including percentage of population with a body mass index (weight/height^2) greater than 30 kg/m^2	
		16.11	Adequate nutrition	Specific recommendations for indicators 16.11 and 16.12 will be submitted to the Regional Committee for approval at the earliest possible opportunity.
		16.12	Exercise	

Target		Regional indicators		
No.	Title	No.	Description	Comment
17	Tobacco, alcohol and psychoactive drugs	17.1	Alcohol consumption	Data from trade publications will be used.
		17.2	Distribution of alcohol consumption by quantity consumed, age and sex	
		17.3	Consumption of the principal narcotic drugs covered by the convention	
		17.4	Mortality from and incidence of homicide and injuries purposely inflicted by other persons (E960-E969)	Source for indicators 17.4 and 17.5 will be routinely reported mortality data.
		17.5	Mortality from certain alcohol-related diseases	
		17.6	Consumption of pharmaceutical psychotropic substances	
		17.7	Number of road traffic accidents involving one or more persons under the influence of alcohol	Information from ECE publications will be used.
		17.8	Use of illicit drugs: – percentages of 15-year-olds who have ever taken an illicit drug and of those who have taken an illicit drug in the last 30 days – number of deaths related to the use of illicit drugs – first admissions for treatment related to drug abuse in a year	

Target		Regional indicators		
No.	Title	No.	Description	Comment
17	Tobacco, alcohol and psychoactive drugs	17.9	Tobacco consumption	Data from *Tobacco journal international* will be used. This is the original indicator 16.1.
		17.10	Proportion of population who: – are nonsmokers – are heavy smokers (20 or more cigarettes per day) – have never smoked – have stopped smoking for the past two years – have reduced smoking for the past two years	Wherever possible, data should be given by sex, age and socioeconomic status. Part of this indicator was the original indicator 16.2. This indicator will also be relevant to target 10.
18	Policy on environment and health		No statistical indicators; narrative situation assessment only.	
19	Environmental health management		No statistical indicators; narrative situation assessment only.	
20	Water quality	20.1	Percentage of the population having access to a sewage system, septic tank or other hygienic means of sewage disposal, separately for urban and rural areas	For indicators 20.1, 20.7, 20.8 and 20.9, data will usually be collated from existing sources.
		20.7	Percentage of the population whose homes are connected to a water supply system, separately for urban and rural areas	
		20.8	Percentage of the population with no access to water within reasonable walking distance	

Target		Regional indicators		
No.	Title	No.	Description	Comment
20	Water quality	20.9	Proportion of the population whose homes are connected to a water supply system ensuring permanent service, with no limitations, throughout the whole year (emergencies and maintenance work excluded)	
		20.10	Proportion of inland surface water meeting national standards for the preparation of drinking-water	Data for indicators 20.10 and 20.11 are available for EC countries.
		20.11	Proportion of recreational water surfaces meeting national standards	
			Percentage of the population whose drinking-water supplies:	
		20.12	are subjected to regular testing of quality, separately for urban and rural areas	
		20.13	meet quality standards applied in regular testing, separately for urban and rural areas	
		20.14	meet WHO 1992 drinking-water quality standards applied in regular testing, separately for urban and rural areas	
21	Air quality	21.4	Number of hours per year in which the average hourly concentration of suspended particulate matter or SO_2 exceeds 250 $\mu g/m^3$ at air quality monitoring stations	

Target		Regional indicators		
No.	Title	No.	Description	Comment
21	Air quality	21.5	Number of hours per year in which the average hourly concentration of ozone exceeds 200 µg/m^3 at air quality monitoring stations	
22	Food quality and safety	22.2	Number and nature of outbreaks of foodborne disease (infections and intoxications) and number of persons involved	Data will be collated from existing sources, where available.
23	Waste management and soil pollution		No statistical indicators; narrative situation assessment only.	
24	Human ecology and settlements	24.3	Proportion of the population that is homeless and proportion of the population that lives in substandard accommodation	
		24.5	Average number of persons per room in occupied housing units and distribution by density, number and percentage	
25	Health of people at work	25.2	Incidence of certified occupational diseases	
		25.4	Working time lost as a result of certified occupational diseases	
		25.5	Percentage of workers exposed at work to average daily noise levels exceeding 90 dBA	
		25.6	Percentage of workers exposed at work to dust levels above recognized standards	

| Target | | Regional indicators | | |
No.	Title	No.	Description	Comment
25	Health of people at work	25.7	Percentage of high-risk workers immunized against hepatitis B	
		25.8	Average number of working days lost per year due to work injuries	
26	Health service policy		No statistical indicators; narrative situation assessment only.	
27	Health service resources and management	27.1	Percentage of total health expenditure devoted to hospital inpatient care	The difference between this percentage and 100% gives a good approximation of expenditure on primary health care. Data for OECD countries are expected to be readily available.
		27.2	Ratio between population and health facilities (primary care units, hospital beds of various types) and personnel (physicians, qualified nurses, auxiliary nursing personnel, midwives, dentists, pharmacists and other trained personnel)	Data reported to and/or collated by WHO will be used.
		27.3	Percentage of physicians and nurses working in hospitals	
		27.4	Percentage of the population covered by public or private insurance funds, by type	
28	Primary health care	28.1	Percentage of infants who by their first birthday have been immunized against diphtheria/pertussis/tetanus (3 doses), poliomyelitis (3 doses), measles (1 dose) and, where required by law, tuberculosis (BCG, I dose); proportion of children immunized against measles before their second birthday, where the country schedule prescribes such immunization	Data reported to and/or collated by WHO will be used.

Target		Regional indicators		
No.	Title	No.	Description	Comment
28	Primary health care	28.5	Number of induced abortions per 1000 live births, by age	If separate rates for the groups aged 0 – 14, 15 – 19 and 20 – 24 years can be identified, these will also be relevant to target 7.
		28.6	Number of live births, by age of mother	Numbers of births to females aged under 16 years, if available, will be relevant to target 7.
29	Hospital care		No statistical indicators; narrative situation assessment only.	
30	Community services to meet special needs		No statistical indicators; narrative situation assessment only.	
31	Quality of care and appropriate technology	31.3	Mortality rates from: – appendicitis (540-543) – hernia and intestinal obstruction (550-553 and 560) – adverse effect of thera-peutic agents (E930-E949)	Source will be routinely reported mortality data.
		31.7	Selected outcome meas-ures for ensuring qual-ity of patient care: – surgical wound infection rates by type of operation – hospital readmission rates – autopsy rates for hospital deaths and all deaths – diabetic complication rates (blindness, nephro-pathy, amputations of (parts of) the extremities, unfavourable pregnancy outcome) – glycated haemoglobin levels	Data on diabetic complications will also be relevant to target 4.
		31.8	Selected process measures for ensuring quality of patient care: – ratio of radiodiagnostic investigations per 1000 population per year – ratio of units of blood transfused per 1000 population per year – ratio of laboratory tests performed per 1000 population per year	

Target		Regional indicators		
No.	Title	No.	Description	Comment
32	Health research and development		No statistical indicators; narrative situation assessment only.	
33	Health for all policy development		No statistical indicators; narrative situation assessment only.	
34	Managing health for all development	34.1	Percentage of the gross national product (GNP) spent on health	
35	Health information support		No statistical indicators; narrative situation assessment only.	
36	Developing human resources for health	36.3	Number of each category of health personnel graduating annually	
37	Partners for health		No statistical indicators; narrative situation assessment only.	
38	Health and ethics		No statistical indicators; narrative situation assessment only.	

Annex 3

Plan of action

**Major events in the monitoring, evaluation and development
of the European health for all (HFA) policy**

Year	Regional Office	Regional Committee (RC)	Member States
1991	Organize analysis of national HFA evaluation reports and draft regional evaluation report on effectiveness of regional strategy and degree to which regional targets have been attained	RC41 to decide on regional report	Report on evaluation of effectiveness of national HFA strategies and degree to which national targets have been attained
	Draft updated version of 1984 regional HFA targets	RC41 to approve updated targets	
1992	Hold expert meetings to put into operation regional indicators on new target areas		
1993	Draft European contribution to Ninth General Programme of Work (GPW) (1996 – 2001)	RC43 to approve regional contribution	

Year	Regional Office	Regional Committee (RC)	Member States
1993 (contd)	Publish updated HFA target book		
	Draft format for regional HFA progress monitoring (including indicators)	RC43 to approve format	
	After RC43, disseminate to Member States integrated global/regional HFA monitoring instrument, accompanied by information available in the Regional Office on selected indicators for updating national reports on the implementation of HFA strategies		Review available HFA monitoring information
1994	Organize a European Conference on Health Policy and Planning – Opportunities for the Future		Participate in Conference
	Prepare summary report on monitoring of implementation of regional HFA strategy, based on information available	RC44 to approve draft regional HFA monitoring report	Submit national HFA monitoring reports
	Organize a Second European Conference on Environment and Health		Participate in Conference
1995	Review epidemiological situation in Europe		
1996	Draft integrated regional/global instrument (with indicators) for HFA evaluation	RC46 to approve instrument and indicators	Start national HFA evaluation

Year	Regional Office	Regional Committee (RC)	Member States
1996 (contd)	After RC46, disseminate to Member States HFA evaluation instrument (with indicators) accompanied by information available in the Regional Office on selected indicators for updating national reports on implementation of HFA strategies		
1997	Organize analysis of national HFA evaluation reports and draft regional report	RC47 to approve regional report	Report on evaluation of effectiveness of national HFA strategies and degree to which national targets have been attained
	Organize consultation with individual Member States and convene workshop on future policy trends in Europe	Regional Health Development Advisory Council to advise on target updating	Advise on need for target updating
1998	Draft updated version of 1991 regional HFA targets	RC48 to approve updated targets	
1999	Draft European contribution to Tenth GPW	RC49 to approve regional contribution	
	Publish updated HFA target book		
	Hold expert meetings to put into operation regional indicators on new target areas and draft format for regional HFA progress monitoring (including indicators)	RC49 to approve format	

Glossary

Appropriate health technology   Methods, procedures, techniques and equipment that are scientifically valid, adapted to local needs, and acceptable to those who use them and to those for whom they are used, and that can be maintained and utilized with resources the community or the country can afford. *(1)*

Community participation   The active involvement of people living together in some form of social organization and cohesion in the planning, operation and control of primary health care, using local, national and other resources. *(1)*

Comprehensive health system   [A health system] that includes all the elements required to meet all the health needs of the population. *(1)*

Disability   In the context of health experience ... any restriction or lack (resulting from an impairment) of ability to perform an activity in the manner or within the range considered normal for a human being. *(2)*

Disease prevention   Measures not only to prevent the occurrence of disease, such as immunization or disease vector control or anti-smoking activities, but also to arrest its progress and reduce its consequences once it is established. *(1)*

Environmental health   Those aspects of human health and disease that are determined by factors in the environment. It also refers to the theory and practice of assessing and controlling factors in the environment that can potentially affect health. Environmental health ... includes both the direct pathological effects of chemicals, radiation and some biological agents, and the effects (often indirect) on health and wellbeing of the broad physical, psychological, social and aesthetic environment, which includes housing, urban development, land use and transport. *(3)*

Equity   Equity in health implies that ideally everyone should have a fair opportunity to attain their full health potential and, more pragmatically, that no one should be disadvantaged from achieving this potential, if it can be avoided. The term *inequity* ... refers to differences in health which are not only unnecessary and avoidable but, in addition, are considered unfair and unjust. *(4)*

Health competence   Individual competence to influence factors determining health. *(5)*

Health for all policy   On the occasion of the thirtieth session of the Regional Committee for Europe at Fez in 1980, representatives of Member States of the WHO European Region approved their first common health policy, the European strategy for attaining health for all. The strategy called for a fundamental change in countries' health development and outlined four main areas of concern: lifestyles and health; risk factors affecting health and the environment; reorientation of the health care system itself; and the political, management, technological, manpower, research and other support necessary to bring about the desired changes in those three areas. In 1991, Member States approved the updated health policy for Europe.

Health for all target   A European (or national) health for all target is a goal towards which to strive in line with the agreed European (or national) health for all policy. It presupposes a political will to commit a country's resources to the achievement of that goal.

Health education   Consciously constructed opportunities for learning which are designed to facilitate changes in behaviour towards a pre-determined goal. *(5)*

Health potential   The fullest degree of health that an individual can achieve. Health potential is determined by caring for oneself and others, by being able to make decisions and take control over one's life, and by ensuring that the society in which one lives creates conditions that allow the attainment of health by all its members.

Health promotion   The process of enabling individuals and communities to increase control over the determinants of health and thereby improve their health. *(5)* An evolving concept that encompasses fostering lifestyles and other social, economic, environmental and personal factors conducive to health. *(1)*

Healthy public policy   An explicit concern for health and equity in all areas of policy and an accountability for health impact. The main aim . . . is to create a supportive environment to enable people to lead healthy lives. *(6)*

Healthy sexuality   Satisfying sexual relations under conditions that preclude contracting sexually transmitted diseases.

Human ecology   A holistic, integrative interpretation of those processes, products, orders and mediating factors that regulate natural and human ecosystems at all scales of the earth's surface and atmosphere. It implies a systemic framework for the analysis and comprehension of three logics and the interrelations between their constituents using a temporal perspective. These three logics are: a bio-logic, or the orders of biological organisms; an eco-logic, or the orders of inorganic constituents (e.g. water, air, soil and sun); a human-logic, or the ordering of cultural, societal and individual human factors. It is suggested that this macro-system of three logics regulates the world. *(7)*

Impairment   In the context of health experience . . . any loss or abnormality of psychological, physiological, or anatomical structure or function. *(2)*

Indicators   Variables that help to measure [changes in the health situation] directly or indirectly and to assess the extent to which the objectives and targets of a programme are being attained. *(1)* For the regional health for all targets, both quantitative and qualitative indicators are used.

Intersectoral action   Action in which the health sector and other relevant sectors collaborate for the achievement of a common goal, the contributions of the different sectors being closely coordinated. *(1)*

Multisectoral action   For practical purposes intersectoral action and multisectoral action are synonymous terms, the former perhaps emphasizing the element of coordination, the latter the contribution of a number of sectors. *(1)*

Parasuicide   An act with nonfatal outcome, in which an individual deliberately initiates a nonhabitual behaviour that, without intervention by others, will cause self-harm, or ingests a substance in excess of the prescribed or generally recognized therapeutic dosage, and which is aimed at realizing changes which he/she desires via the actual or expected physical consequences. *(8)*

Primary care   The first level of care, generally provided in an ambulatory setting (as opposed to secondary and tertiary care which would normally be hospital-based).

Primary health care   Essential health care made accessible at a cost the country and community can afford, with methods that are practical, scientifically sound and socially acceptable. Primary health care is the central function and main focus of a country's health system, the principal vehicle for the delivery of health care, the most peripheral level in a health system stretching from the periphery to the centre, and an integral part of the social and economic development of a country. *(1)*

Quality of care   The extent to which the care provided, within a given economic framework, achieves the most favourable outcome when balancing risks and benefits.

Quality of life   The perception of individuals or groups that their needs are being satisfied and that they are not being denied opportunities to achieve happiness and fulfilment. *(5)*

Secondary care   Referral services in the first instance provide secondary health care, which is of a more specialized kind than can be offered at the most peripheral level, for example radiographic diagnosis, general surgery, care of women with complications of pregnancy or childbirth, and diagnosis and treatment of uncommon or severe diseases. This kind of care is provided by trained staff in such institutions as district or provincial hospitals. *(1)*

Social marginalization   The process by which certain vulnerable groups may be prevented from participating fully in social, political and economic life in a community. This occurs when the necessary intersectoral policies and support mechanisms are not in place to enable their full participation.

Strategy   A long-term considered and comprehensive course of action that provides the framework for individual activities and events.

Supportive environments   In a health context ... both the physical and the social aspects of our surroundings. It encompasses where people live, their local community, their home, where they work and play. It also embraces the framework which determines access to resources for living, and opportunities for empowerment. Thus action to create supportive environments has many dimensions: physical, social, spiritual, economic and political. Each of these dimensions is inextricably linked to the others in a dynamic interaction. *(9)*

Tertiary care   Specialized care that requires highly specific facilities and the attention of highly specialized health workers, for example, for neurosurgery or heart surgery. *(1)*

Sources of definitions

1. *Glossary of terms used in the "Health for All" Series, No. 1 – 8*. Geneva, World Health Organization, 1984 ("Health for all" Series, No. 9).
2. *International Classification of Impairments, Disabilities, and Handicaps*. Geneva, World Health Organization, 1980.
3. *Environment and health. The European Charter and commentary*. Copenhagen, WHO Regional Office for Europe, 1990 (WHO Regional Publications, European Series, No. 35).
4. WHITEHEAD, M. *The concepts and principles of equity and health*. Copenhagen, WHO Regional Office for Europe, 1990 (document EUR/ICP/RPD 414).
5. *Health promotion glossary*. Copenhagen, WHO Regional Office for Europe, 1989 (document).
6. The Adelaide recommendations: healthy public policy. *Health promotion*, **3**: 183 – 186 (1988).
7. Human ecology and environmental policies: prospects for politics and planning. *Political geography quarterly*, **9**: 103 – 107 (1990).
8. *Working group on preventive practices in suicide and attempted suicide*. Copenhagen, WHO Regional Office for Europe, 1986 (document EUR/ICP/PSF 017(S)).
9. *Sundsvall Statement on Supportive Environments for Health*. Third International Conference on Health Promotion, Sundsvall, Sweden, 9 – 15 June 1991. Geneva, World Health Organization, 1991 (document WHO/HED/92.1)

Index of subjects